Personalized Medicine in Ophthalmic Diseases: Challenges and Opportunities

Personalized Medicine in Ophthalmic Diseases: Challenges and Opportunities

Editors

Kai Jin
Chun Zhang

MDPI • Basel • Beijing • Wuhan • Barcelona • Belgrade • Manchester • Tokyo • Cluj • Tianjin

Editors
Kai Jin
Zhejiang University
Hangzhou, China

Chun Zhang
Peking University Third Hospital
Beijing, China

Editorial Office
MDPI
St. Alban-Anlage 66
4052 Basel, Switzerland

This is a reprint of articles from the Special Issue published online in the open access journal *Journal of Personalized Medicine* (ISSN 2075-4426) (available at: https://www.mdpi.com/journal/jpm/special_issues/5A4T9V0J0V).

For citation purposes, cite each article independently as indicated on the article page online and as indicated below:

LastName, A.A.; LastName, B.B.; LastName, C.C. Article Title. *Journal Name* **Year**, *Volume Number*, Page Range.

ISBN 978-3-0365-8020-3 (Hbk)
ISBN 978-3-0365-8021-0 (PDF)

Contents

About the Editors

Kai Jin

Prof. Kai Jin is a doctor and research scientist of the Department of Ophthalmology, the Second Affiliated hospital of Zhejiang University School of Medicine. His current research interests are as follows: retina, imaging, artificial intelligence, and personalized medicine. He received his PhD in 2018 and has an outstanding publication record, with 50 publications in peer-reviewed international journals, and his google scholar citations number is 909. In the past year, Dr. Jin has been awarded the WILEY Top Cited Article Award. According to 2023 data from the Expertscape, he ranks 0.39% of the global top in the field of deep learning research.

Chun Zhang

Chun Zhang is a professor and former honorary professor of the Department of Ophthalmology of the University of Hong Kong. He is currently the Director of the Glaucoma Service of the Third Hospital of Peking University, and the Director of the Beijing Key Laboratory for Reconstruction, Protection, and Rehabilitation of Ocular Nerve Injuries. He also has many academic contributions, including being a national member of the Ophthalmology Society of the Chinese Medical Association and a member of the Chinese Glaucoma Society, as well as a member of many international academic organizations. Has won the Achievement Award of the APAO and the Second Prize of the Beijing Science and Technology Progress Award.

Journal of
Personalized
Medicine

MDPI

Editorial

Personalized Medicine in Ophthalmic Diseases: Challenges and Opportunities

Kai Jin [1,*] and Chun Zhang [2,*]

1 Eye Center, The Second Affiliated Hospital, School of Medicine, Zhejiang University, Hangzhou 310009, China
2 Department of Ophthalmology, Peking University Third Hospital, Beijing 100191, China
* Correspondence: jinkai@zju.edu.cn (K.J.); zhangc1@yahoo.com (C.Z.)

Citation: Jin, K.; Zhang, C. Personalized Medicine in Ophthalmic Diseases: Challenges and Opportunities. *J. Pers. Med.* **2023**, *13*, 893. https://doi.org/10.3390/jpm13060893

Received: 23 May 2023
Accepted: 23 May 2023
Published: 25 May 2023

1. Introduction

Personalized medicine is a broadly used term to encompass approaches used to tailor healthcare to the needs of individual patients [1]. It can lead to more effective treatments for patients in ophthalmology, reducing the need for trial-and-error approaches and potentially avoiding unnecessary treatments. This can also lead to cost savings for healthcare systems. Diagnostic techniques that can realize comprehensive individual assessment are important. Next-generation sequencing and translational research are some of the techniques put forward by previous studies. Gene therapy-based treatment trials have been presented for ophthalmic diseases, such as retinitis pigmentosa and age-related macular degeneration.

2. The Role of Artificial Intelligence and Telemedicine in Diagnostic Techniques

Recently, with the rapid development of Artificial Intelligence and interdisciplinary collaboration, concepts like machine learning and wearable device have been frequently raised in ophthalmic research [2]. There might be new promising methods to realize personalized ophthalmology. The ophthalmology field was among the first to adopt Artificial Intelligence (AI) in medicine. The availability of digitized ocular images and substantial data have made deep learning (DL) a popular topic. At the moment, AI in ophthalmology is mostly used to improve disease diagnosis and assist decision-making in ophthalmic diseases such as diabetic retinopathy (DR), glaucoma, age-related macular degeneration (AMD), cataract and other anterior segment diseases. However, most of the AI systems developed to date are still in the experimental stages, with only a few having achieved clinical applications. There are a number of reasons for this phenomenon, including security, privacy, poor pervasiveness, trust and explainability concerns [3]. Telemedicine screening needs to be tailored to the targeted population in order to reap the benefits of digital technology.

3. Gene Therapy-Based Treatment and Personalized Medicine

Recent developments in the field of gene therapy have attracted interest from scientists, clinicians and industry. Gene therapy approaches with the most promise in terms of visual improvements and longevity can be determined with the help of retinal and deep phenotyping. Progress in genotyping techniques and back-of-the-eye scans are helping us understand the diseases and their manifestations in patients. The majority of vision loss in diseases of the eye is caused by the loss of photoreceptor function. The appropriate therapeutic approach to use for each patient is determined by the timing and circumstances surrounding the loss of photoreceptor function. Gene therapy is rapidly becoming a therapeutic reality in the clinic. The move from laboratory work to clinical application has been propelled by advances in our understanding of disease genetics and mechanisms [4]. The beginning of the twenty-first century was marked by the innovative use of pharmacochemical interventions. One of the first applications of novel genome editing technologies was the treatment of rare inherited retinopathies. A new era of precision medicine will be ushered in by the exciting development of newer, cutting-edge strategies including base editing and prime editing [5].

4. Challenges and Opportunities

AI coupled with teleophthalmology presents an opportunity to promote equity in eye health [6]. It is indicated that novel screening strategies, such as AI-based screening, could achieve greater cost-effectiveness in population screening. Routine screening for multiple blindness-causing eye diseases could be highly cost-effective in China, providing robust economic evidence for informed policy making regarding its large-scale promotion. Although ophthalmic AI and telemedicine show promise for patients, there are significant barriers to widespread adoption. Clinicians will be tasked with embracing innovation while ensuring protocols and implementation are evidence-based and improve outcomes [7]. Interpretability and expandability are crucial factors in AI-based medical screening systems. Interpretability refers to the ability of the system to provide clear and understandable explanations for its decisions, which is important for gaining the trust of medical professionals and patients. Expandability refers to the ability of the system to adapt and improve over time as new data become available [8].

The first successful implementation of AAV-mediated gene augmentation therapy is for the treatment of retinitis pigmentosa, a dozen other clinical trials are underway to tackle other monogenic diseases of the retina using this strategy [4]. Gene therapy still has a negative effect on the eye. Different cell types require different gene therapies. The cost of clinical trials will likely be reduced in the years to come as a result of this and anticipated developments in the manufacturing practices of core technologies. In the years to come, methods to safely and specifically edit the genes are likely to be crucial. Due to the complexity of silence and replacement strategies, clinical trials have not been able to target the autosomal-dominant genes causing retinal degeneration. Future developments in the evaluation of low vision along with development of more sophisticated instruments for objective measures is going to be key to the achievement of such therapies.

Author Contributions: Conceptualization, K.J. and C.Z.; writing—original draft preparation, K.J.; writing—review and editing, C.Z. All authors have read and agreed to the published version of the manuscript.

Conflicts of Interest: The authors declare no conflict of interest.

References

1. Yamamoto, Y.; Kanayama, N.; Nakayama, Y.; Matsushima, N. Current Status, Issues and Future Prospects of Personalized Medicine for Each Disease. *J. Pers. Med.* **2022**, *12*, 444. [CrossRef] [PubMed]
2. Li, J.O.; Liu, H.; Ting, D.S.J.; Jeon, S.; Chan, R.V.P.; Kim, J.E.; Sim, D.A.; Thomas, P.B.M.; Lin, H.; Chen, Y.; et al. Digital technology, tele-medicine and artificial intelligence in ophthalmology: A global perspective. *Prog. Retin. Eye Res.* **2021**, *82*, 100900. [CrossRef] [PubMed]
3. Jin, K.; Ye, J. Artificial intelligence and deep learning in ophthalmology: Current status and future perspectives. *Adv. Ophthalmol. Pract. Res.* **2022**, *2*, 100078. [CrossRef]
4. Botto, C.; Rucli, M.; Tekinsoy, M.D.; Pulman, J.; Sahel, J.A.; Dalkara, D. Early and late stage gene therapy interventions for inherited retinal degenerations. *Prog. Retin. Eye Res.* **2022**, *86*, 100975. [CrossRef] [PubMed]
5. Levi, S.R.; Ryu, J.; Liu, P.K.; Tsang, S.H. Precision Medicine Trials in Retinal Degenerations. *Annu. Rev. Vis. Sci.* **2021**, *7*, 851–865. [CrossRef] [PubMed]
6. Liu, H.; Li, R.; Zhang, Y.; Zhang, K.; Yusufu, M.; Liu, Y.; Mou, D.; Chen, X.; Tian, J.; Li, H.; et al. Economic evaluation of combined population-based screening for multiple blindness-causing eye diseases in China: A cost-effectiveness analysis. *Lancet Glob. Health* **2023**, *11*, e456–e465. [CrossRef]
7. Rathi, S.; Tsui, E.; Mehta, N.; Zahid, S.; Schuman, J.S. The Current State of Teleophthalmology in the United States. *Ophthalmology* **2017**, *124*, 1729–1734. [CrossRef] [PubMed]
8. Cao, J.; You, K.; Zhou, J.; Xu, M.; Xu, P.; Wen, L.; Wang, S.; Jin, K.; Lou, L.; Wang, Y.; et al. A cascade eye diseases screening system with interpretability and expandability in ultra-wide field fundus images: A multicentre diagnostic accuracy study. *eClinicalMedicine* **2022**, *53*, 101633. [CrossRef] [PubMed]

Journal of *Personalized Medicine*

MDPI

Article

Analysis of Clinical Characteristics of Patients with Recurrent Cytomegalovirus Retinitis after Hematopoietic Stem Cell Transplantation

Xiaona Wang †, Yao Lu †, Haiping Li, Zhizhong Ma, Jing Hong and Changguan Wang *

Department of Ophthalmology, Beijing Key Laboratory of Restoration of Damaged Ocular Nerve, Peking University Third Hospital, Beijing 100191, China; 15801635367@163.com (X.W.); hongjing196401@163.com (J.H.)
* Correspondence: bysyeyecenter@163.com; Tel.: +86-010-8226-6359
† These authors contributed equally to this work.

Abstract: Objective: To analyze and summarize the clinical and imaging characteristics of patients with cytomegalovirus retinitis (CMVR) relapse after hematopoietic stem cell transplantation (HSCT). Methods: This retrospective case series study recruited patients with CMVR after HSCT. The study compared the patients with stable lesions and CMV-negative aqueous humor after treatment with those with relapse lesions and a CMV DNA load in aqueous humor which had increased again after treatment. The observation indexes were basic clinical information, best-corrected visual acuity, wide-angle fundus photography, optical coherence tomography (OCT), blood $CD4^+$ T lymphocyte count, and aqueous humor CMV load of the patients. We summarized the data and statistically analyzed the differences between the relapse and non-relapse groups, as well as the correlations of the observed indicators. Results: The study recruited 52 patients with CMVR (82 eyes) after HSCT, of whom 11 patients (15 eyes) had recurrence after treatment (21.2%). The recurrence interval was 6.4 ± 4.9 months. The final best-corrected visual acuity of recurrent patients was 0.3 ± 0.3. The number of $CD4^+$ T lymphocytes in recurrence patients at the time of onset was $126.7 \pm 80.2/\text{mm}^3$. The median CMV DNA load detected in aqueous humor at the time of recurrence was 8.63×10^3 copies/mL. There was a significant difference in the $CD4^+$ T lymphocyte count between the recurrence and the non-recurrence groups at onset. The onset of visual acuity in recurrence patients was significantly correlated with final visual acuity and recurrence lesion area. The fundus of recurred CMVR showed increased marginal activity of the original stable lesion. Concurrently, yellow-white new lesions appeared around the stable, atrophic, and necrotic lesions. OCT showed new diffuse hyperreflexic lesions in the retinal neuroepithelial layer near the old lesions. Inflammatory punctate hyperreflexes were observed in the vitreous, with vitreous liquefaction and contraction. Conclusion: This study suggests that the clinical features, fundus manifestations, and imaging features of CMVR recurrence after HSCT are different from those at the initial onset. Patients should be closely followed up after their condition is stable to be alert for CMVR recurrence.

Keywords: hematopoietic stem cell transplantation; cytomegalovirus retinitis; recurrence; wide-angle fundus photography; optical coherence tomography; polymerase chain reaction; CD4

Citation: Wang, X.; Lu, Y.; Li, H.; Ma, Z.; Hong, J.; Wang, C. Analysis of Clinical Characteristics of Patients with Recurrent Cytomegalovirus Retinitis after Hematopoietic Stem Cell Transplantation. *J. Pers. Med.* **2023**, *13*, 639. https://doi.org/10.3390/jpm13040639

Academic Editors: Ana Isabel Ramírez Sebastián, Kai Jin and Chun Zhang

Received: 10 February 2023
Revised: 17 March 2023
Accepted: 23 March 2023
Published: 7 April 2023

1. Introduction

Cytomegalovirus (CMV) infection remains an important cause of morbidity and mortality in patients who undergo hematopoietic stem cell transplantation HSCT, because the estimated seroprevalence for blood and organ donors is 90% in China [1–4]. Cytomegalovirus retinitis (CMVR) is the most common fundus disease in people with low immune function [5–8]. Typical fundus manifestations of the disease are yellow-white fusion lesions that progress along the retinal vessels, accompanied by retinal hemorrhage and edema, showing a typical "cheese and tomato sauce" appearance. Systemic and intravitreal injections of ganciclovir have become a recognized method of treatment of CMVR [9].

However, in clinical practice, we found that patients with different immune reconstitution statuses after HSCT had different disease outcomes. Not all CMVR lesions are stable and can be maintained after aqueous humor polymerase chain reaction (PCR) detection turns negative. In recent years, domestic and foreign literature has gradually paid increased attention to the diagnosis and treatment of CMVR after HSCT; however, there are no reports on the clinical characteristics and imaging manifestations of patients with recurrence after CMVR treatment and HSCT. Therefore, this study analyzed and summarized the clinical characteristics and imaging changes in these patients, aiming to provide a basis for optimization of the diagnosis and treatment of CMVR after HSCT.

2. Materials and Methods

2.1. Data Collection

This retrospective case series study included patients who were diagnosed with CMVR after HSCT and recurrence after treatment at the Ophthalmology Center of Peking University Third Hospital from January 2018 to October 2022. Inclusion criteria: (1) History of HSCT; (2) CMVR diagnosis according to typical fundus manifestations and positive CMV DNA in aqueous humor with deoxyribonucleic acid (DNA) PCR testing; (3) Patients whose previous CMVR lesions were stable and aqueous humor CMV DNA was negative, who showed a recurrent CMVR lesion and recurrence of aqueous humor CMV DNA positivity. Exclusion criteria: Patients with a history of other systemic and eye diseases, who had undergone other eye surgery or laser treatment in the past, and who could not cooperate with regular follow-up and treatment, were excluded from the study. This study was approved by the Ethics Committee of Peking University Third Hospital. Ethics approval number: 2015; Medical Ethics Review number: 197. The study followed the principles of the Declaration of Helsinki.

The medical history and basic information of the enrolled patients were collected, including gender, age, primary disease, affected eyes, date of hematopoietic stem cell transplantation, date of ocular onset, date of ocular recurrence, peripheral blood $CD4^{+}$ T lymphocyte count, and the results of ocular aqueous humor virus examination at the time of recurrence. The CMV DNA in aqueous humor was detected by PCR, and the $CD4^{+}$ T lymphocyte count in the patients was detected by flow cytometry.

Follow-up observation was carried out on the CMVR lesions of the patients. CMVR lesion locations were divided into 3 zones: zone 1 consisted of the area within 3000 mm of the center of the macula (macular involvement) or within 1500 mm of the margin of the optic disc (disc involvement), zone 2 consisted of the area anterior to zone 1 to the equator, and zone 3 consisted of the area anterior to zone 2 to the ora serrata [5]. Image J software was used to measure the lesion and optic disc areas of the patients with recurrence, and the ratio of the lesion area to optic disc area was recorded.

2.2. Follow-Up and Treatment Plan

After the initial diagnosis of CMVR, all patients underwent regular intravitreal antiviral therapy until the lesion was completely stable and CMV DNA tests of the aqueous humor were negative. Thereafter, the patients were followed up once a month for the required eye examinations, including best-corrected visual acuity (BCVA), intraocular pressure, slit lamp examination, ophthalmoscopy after mydriasis, wide-angle fundus photography (Optos PLC, Dunfermline, UK), and optical coherence tomography (Heidelberg Engineering, Heidelberg, Germany). According to the fundus examination, if the lesions were suspected to have recurred, PCR testing of the aqueous humor was performed to confirm CMVR recurrence, and the antiviral treatment was reinitiated.

All patients were administered an intravitreal injection of ganciclovir immediately after the CMVR diagnosis was confirmed. The dosage of ganciclovir was 3 mg/0.1 mL by intravitreal injection. During the induction period, the intravitreal injection was administered twice a week for 2 weeks. The maintenance period was once a week until the lesion became stable and the viral load of the aqueous humor turned negative. For systemic antiviral treatment, the hematologist in charge adjusted the drug regimen according to the systemic CMV infection, and regularly monitored the liver and kidney functions. For the patients with CMVR recurrence, intravitreal injections of ganciclovir were reinitiated. For the patients with poor response of fundus lesions after treatment, intravitreal injections of ganciclovir were combined with foscarnet sodium.

2.3. Statistical Analysis

SPSS software (version 24.0, Chicago, IL, USA) was used for statistical analysis. Descriptive data were recorded as mean ± standard deviation. *t*-tests and chi-squared tests were used to analyze the differences between groups, and Pearson's correlation analysis was used to analyze the correlations. A p-value < 0.05 was considered statistically significant.

3. Results

3.1. Basic Data

During the follow-up period, the research team collected data on 52 cases (82 eyes) of CMVR after HSCT; these included 32 male (61.5%) and 20 female patients (38.5%). Of the 52 cases, 21 were monocular and 31 were binocular. The average age of patients was 27.0 ± 15.4 years (4–71 years). The best-corrected visual acuity of all patients at onset was 0.50 ± 0.39 (HM–1.0, LogMAR visual acuity: 0.71), and the best-corrected visual acuity of all patients at the treatment end point was 0.46 ± 0.36 (HM–1.0, LogMAR visual acuity: 0.69).

During the follow-up, 11 patients had recurrence during treatment, for a total of 15 eyes (recurrence rate: 21.2%). The recurrent patients included five males (45.5%) and six females (54.5%), with an average age of 30.3 ± 21.8 years (7–65 years), of which seven cases were monocular and four cases were binocular. The interval between recurrence and first onset was 6.4 ± 4.9 months (1–18 months). The initial best-corrected visual acuity of the patients with recurrence was 0.5 ± 0.4 (0.05–1.0, LogMAR visual acuity: 0.3). The best-corrected visual acuity record of the recurrent patients after treatment was 0.3 ± 0.3 (HM–1.0, LogMAR visual acuity: 0.5).

There was a significant difference between the recurrence and non-recurrence groups in the blood CD4 lymphocyte count at the onset. Other indicators, including gender ratio, unilateral and bilateral incidence ratio, onset age, initial visual acuity, final visual acuity, and viral load showed no statistical difference between groups (Table 1). The initial visual acuity of the recurrence patients was significantly correlated with recurrent visual acuity ($p < 0.05$, correlation coefficient 0.844). The patient's visual acuity at the time of recurrence decreased significantly ($p = 0.001$). The correlation analysis of the visual acuity of the recurrence patients at onset and the lesion area at the time of recurrence had $p = 0.064$, and a correlation coefficient of −0.49 (Tables 2 and 3).

3.2. CD4⁺ T Lymphocyte Count

The peripheral blood $CD4^+$ T lymphocyte count of all CMVR patients at the time of onset was 133 ± 67.5/mm^3 (40–320/mm^3). The average $CD4^+$ T lymphocyte count of the recurrent CMVR patients was 129.7 ± 80.7/mm^3 (30–288/mm^3). The number of $CD4^+$ T lymphocytes in blood was less than 50/mm^3 in one case of recurrence, less than 200/mm^3 in eight cases, and more than 200/mm^3 in two cases. The $CD4^+$ T lymphocyte count had no correlation with age of onset, recurrence interval, initial visual acuity, visual acuity at recurrence, viral load in aqueous humor at recurrence, and lesion area at recurrence.

Table 1. Comparison of clinical data between recurrent and non-recurrent CMVR patients after HSCT.

Group	Number of People/Eye	Male /Female	Unilateral /Bilateral	Age (Years)	Onset Visual Acuity	Final Visual Acuity	Viral Load (Copies/mL)	Onset CD4 Count (/mm^3)
Non recurrent group	41/67	27/14	14/27	26.0 ± 13.4	0.5 ± 0.4	0.5 ± 0.4	4.17×10^3	295.7 ± 171.7
Recurrent group	11/15	5/6	7/4	30.3 ± 21.8	0.5 ± 0.4	0.3 ± 0.3	8.63×10^3	129.7 ± 80.7
Total	52/82	32/20	21/31	27.0 ± 15.4	0.5 ± 0.4	0.5 ± 0.4	7.18×10^3	243.6 ± 168.1
***p*-Value**	/	0.22	0.08	0.54	0.42	0.68	0.57	**0.00**

Table 2. Clinical information of patients with recurrent CMVR after HSCT.

Number	Gender	Age	Eye	Recurrence Interval (M)	Initial Visual Acuity	Recurrent Visual Acuity	$CD4^+$ T Lymphocyte Count at Recurrence (/mm^3)	Viral Load at Recurrence (Copies/mL)	Lesion Area at Recurrence (PD)	Recurrence Causes	Primary Disease
1	Male	7	Left	1	0.05	HM	191	1.08×10^3	226.7	Immune hemolysis	ALL
2	Male	47	Left	5	0.1	0.05	288	1.30×10^2	25.2	Persistent viremia	AML
			Right	6	0.6	0.05		3.29×10^4	20.6		
3	Male	8	Right	5	0.6	0.5	30	6.42×10^2	30	Liver rejection	MDS
4	Female	10	Left	14	0.3	0.1	94	1.35×10^4	23.1	Liver rejection	AA
			Right	13	0.5	0.3		8.63×10^3	77.3		
5	Female	10	Left	3	0.8	0.5	56	1.24×10^3	65.2	Liver and intestinal rejection	MDS
6	Male	51	Right	3	0.5	0.2	72	2.08×10^4	130.7	Liver and skin rejection	AML
7	Female	65	Right	3	1	0.3	105	4.36×10^3	7.8	Age related immunosuppression	CML
8	Female	32	Left	9	0.3	0.1	195	3.07×10^7	41.3	Continuous decrease in $CD4^+$ T lymphocyte count	ALL
9	Female	58	Right	18	0.6	0.12	122	2.57×10^5	18.3	Liver and Lung rejection	AML
10	Female	16	Left	3	0.5	0.3	62	2.23×10^2	90.8	Skin rejection	ALL
			Right	3	0.05	0.05		8.99×10^2	129.7		
11	Male	29	Left	5	1	1	212	1.39×10^4	43.1	Liver rejection	AML
			Right	5	0.5	0.5		4.46×10^4	8.8		

ALL Acute lymphoblastic leukemia; AML Acute myeloid leukemia; AA Aplastic anemia; MDS Myelodysplastic syndrome; CML Chronic myeloid leukemia.

Table 3. Statistical table of clinical data of patients with recurrent CMVR after HSCT.

Index		Age	Recurrence Interval	Initial Visual Acuity	CD4+ T Lymphocyte Count at Recurrence	Viral Load at Recurrence	Recurrent Visual Acuity	Lesion Area at Recurrence
Age	CC	/	0.106	0.316	0.367	0.045	0.079	−0.411
	P		0.707	0.251	0.178	0.873	0.78	0.128
Recurrence interval	CC	0.106	/	0.002	−0.024	0.152	−0.232	−0.436
	P	0.707		0.995	0.932	0.589	0.405	0.104
Initial visual acuity	CC	0.316	0.002	/	−0.15	−0.177	0.844	−0.49
	P	0.251	0.995		0.594	0.528	0	0.064
CD4+ T lymphocyte count at recurrence	CC	0.367	−0.024	−0.15	/	0.183	−0.148	−0.203
	P	0.178	0.932	0.594		0.514	0.598	0.469
Viral load at recurrence	CC	0.045	0.152	−0.177	0.183	/	−0.19	−0.099
	P	0.873	0.589	0.528	0.514		0.497	0.725
Recurrent visual acuity	CC	0.079	−0.232	0.844	−0.148	−0.19	/	−0.356
	P	0.78	0.405	0	0.598	0.497		0.193
Lesion area at recurrence	CC	−0.411	−0.436	−0.49	−0.203	−0.099	−0.356	/
	P	0.128	0.104	0.064	0.469	0.725	0.193	
	Mean	30.3	6.4	0.5	129.7	2073327	0.3	62.6
	SD	21.8	4.9	0.3	80.7	7919595	0.3	60.7

3.3. Detection of Viral Load in Aqueous Humor

The CMV load at the onset of all patients was 0 to 6.64×10^7 copies/mL, median 7.18×10^3 copies/mL. The viral load of the recurrent patients was 2.23×10^2 to 3.07×10^7 copies/mL, median 8.63×10^3 copies/mL. Among them, four eyes had $<1 \times 10^3$ copies/mL, nine had $>1 \times 10^3$ and $<1 \times 10^5$ copies/mL, and the CMV DNA load of two eyes was $>1 \times 10^5$ copies/mL. There was no significant correlation between the viral load in aqueous humor of the recurrent patients and age of onset, recurrence interval, initial visual acuity, visual acuity at recurrence, $CD4^+$ T lymphocyte count at recurrence, and lesion area at recurrence.

3.4. Characteristics of Fundus Lesions

After recurrence, nine eyes had fundus lesions in zone 1, eight had simultaneous optic disc and macula involvement (average visual acuity: 0.25), and one had mainly optic disc involvement. Two eyes had lesions in zone 2, one eye on the nasal side of the optic disc, and one on the temporal side of the vascular arch. One eye had lesions in zone 3. ImageJ software was used to measure the lesion and optic disc area of the recurrent patients, and the ratio of the lesion to optic disc area was recorded. The average lesion size was 62.6 ± 60.7 optic disc areas of the recurrent patients, including three eyes with >100 optic disc areas, ten eyes with >10 optic disc areas <100 optic disc areas, and two eyes with <10 optic disc areas. Recurrent fundus mainly manifested as a new yellowish fusion focus surrounding the original atrophic area, or a new small cluster of yellowish-white lesions, which may be accompanied by retinal vasculitis (Figure 1). Eight eyes had lesions involving the optic disc and macula simultaneously, one eye had retinal neovascularization, two eyes had retinal and inferior fiber proliferation, and three eyes had obvious vitreous inflammatory opacity.

The p-value of the correlation analysis between the lesion area and the initial visual acuity was 0.064, and the correlation coefficient was −0.49. The lesion area at recurrence was not related to the age of onset, recurrence interval, visual acuity at recurrence, $CD4^+$ T lymphocyte count at recurrence, or viral load in aqueous humor at recurrence.

3.5. OCT Features

The OCT image of the lesion area was analyzed and described, with the scanning scope covering the original necrotic focus and the marginal recurrent focus. OCT images of recurrent lesions mainly showed diffuse hyperreflexes in the retinal neuroepithelial layer, blurred retinal layers, microcavity formation, cystoid edema within retinal layers, and exudative detachment of the retinal neuroepithelial layer, with punctate hyperreflexes in the vitreous body. During the observation and follow-up of these patients, OCT also detected liquefaction and contraction of the vitreous body due to inflammatory stimulation, as well as separation of the retinal inner limiting membrane and the vitreous posterior limiting membrane (Figure 2). Eight eyes of the enrolled patients showed punctate hyperreflexes of the vitreous body accompanied by traction of the posterior limiting membrane, and one eye showed retinal breaks on scanning. Among them, one eye underwent vitrectomy combined with silicone oil tamponade due to retinal detachment, and three eyes underwent vitrectomy to remove traction due to the aggravation of retinal proliferation.

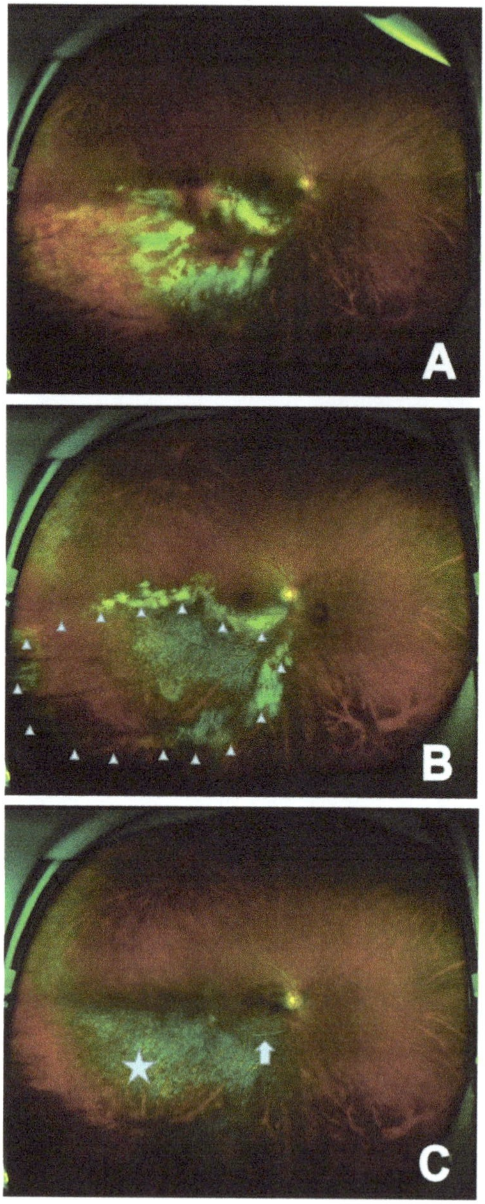

Figure 1. In the right eye of case 6, the lesion appears as fulminant/edematous type. The onset focus of the fundus showed a yellow-white patchy fusion lesion that had formed in the infratemporal branch of the retina with development of retinal hemorrhage (**A**); recurrent fundus mainly manifests as new yellow-white fusion around the original atrophic area (△) (**B**); the stable focus showed gray atrophy of retina (☆) with local retinal artery occlusion (↑) (**C**).

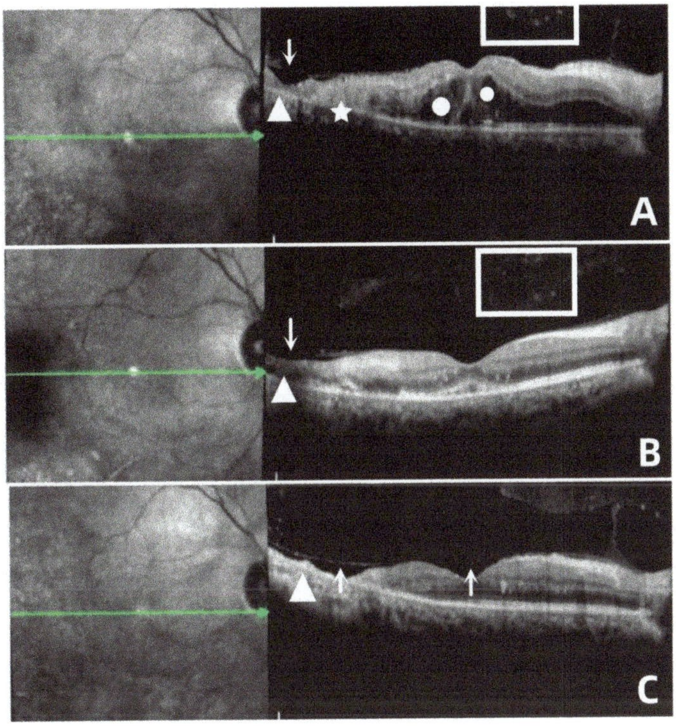

Figure 2. (**A**) In case 6, the recurrent focus was located at the edge of the atrophic focus (△), showing diffuse hyperreflexes (☆) across the whole layer of the retina, accompanied by multiple punctate hyperreflexes in the vitreous body (□) and macular edema (○), as well as disorder of the outer layer of the retina. (**B**) Retinal edema gradually subsided; small cavities (↓) were formed in the necrotic area, and the outer structure of retina was partially repaired after antiviral treatment. (**C**) Stable lesions showed retinal atrophy with choroidal atrophy (△), vitreous liquefaction and contraction, and separation of the inner limiting membrane and vitreous posterior limiting membrane (↑).

4. Discussion

Cytomegalovirus retinitis is the most common opportunistic ocular infection in people with low immune function. The fundus mainly shows yellow-white granular fusion lesions with hemorrhage, accompanied by vitreous inflammation and retinal vasculitis, showing typical "cheese and tomato sauce" changes. Those most commonly affected are patients with AIDS and HSCT [10–12]. In recent years, many reports have been published on CMVR in patients with AIDS, but reports on CMVR after HSCT are limited, and the clinical characteristics of patients with CMVR recurrence after HSCT have not been reported.

There are many reasons for CMVR recurrence after HSCT, among which two key factors are the $CD4^+$ T lymphocyte count and the CMV load in aqueous humor.

With regard to the $CD4^+$ T lymphocyte count, the literature showed that the T lymphocyte subsets were significantly lower in CMVR cases within six months after HSCT (all $p < 0.05$) [13]. CMVR often occurs in patients whose $CD4^+$ T lymphocyte count is less than $50/mm^3$ [6,14]. CMVR occurred more often among the recipients from alternative donors. The risk of viral infections is higher in HSCT from alternative donors including haploidentical donors and unrelated donors than human leukocyte antigen-matched sibling donors due to their severely depressed T cell-mediated immune response and insufficient resistance to the virus [15–18]. We found that the average $CD4^+$ T lymphocyte count in the patients with recurrent CMVR after HSCT was significantly higher than the reference values provided in previous studies. The CD4$^+$ T lymphocyte count in the recurrent group was significantly lower than that in the non-recurrent group. (1) These data show that even if the immune status of HSCT patients is not very poor, it is still possible to have a recurrence of ocular CMVR. Even if the number of CD4$^+$ T lymphocytes has exceeded 200/mm^3, stricter, more regular follow-ups should be carried out and the antiviral treatment should be supplemented in time according to the actual conditions of the patient. (2) The expert consensus on AIDS combined with CMVR treatment suggests that, if the CD4$^+$ T lymphocyte count is 50–100/mm^3, the fundus examination frequency should be once every three months and once every 6–12 months for those with a CD4$^+$ T lymphocyte count greater than 100/mm^3 [19]. This follow-up density is slightly insufficient for observing CMVR recurrence after HSCT. This study advocates that within six months after the first stabilization of CMVR in HSCT patients, the CMVR should be rechecked every 1–3 months in combination with individual immune status, and every three months from 6–12 months after the stabilization of CMVR. (3) This article summarizes the possible causes of immunosuppression in patients with CMVR recurrence after HSCT, such as immunological hemolysis and continuous multiple organ rejection. Six patients with CMVR recurrence after HSCT had a liver rejection. The existing literature also suggests that patients with liver rejection after HSCT are more likely to develop acute graft versus host reaction and have greater immune damage [19]. Acute and chronic graft versus host disease (GVHD) has been identified as an independent risk factor for the development of CMVR after HSCT for primary immunodeficiency and hematological disorders [20]. Patients with CMVR recurrence after HSCT experience more specificity in systemic and local inflammatory reactions and immune status [21]. We cannot simply follow the clinical experience of HSCT patients with CMVR at the first onset [22,23]. We should pay close attention to the changes in the disease and treat it with caution.

The CMV load in aqueous humor is also an important reason for CMVR recurrence in HSCT patients, and there is a linear relationship between the CMV load and the active lesion area of CMVR (the CMV load in aqueous humor = 3.38 + 0.01 × active lesion area) [6]. For patients with CMVR recurrence after HSCT, the CMV DNA load in aqueous humor varies greatly (10^2 to 10^7 copies/mL). The viral load in aqueous humor in three patients was less than 10^3 copies/mL when they relapsed. Therefore, the definition of 10^3 copies/mL as the standard for stopping treatment in some literature was also slightly inappropriate [16,17,24]. According to our results, even if the lesions of the CMVR patients after HSCT are completely stable and the CMV DNA in the eyes is completely negative, a considerable number of patients will still have CMVR lesion recurrence. From systemic virus infection, research indicated that even after the status of CMV antigenemia-negative had been achieved, active CMV infection remained in the retina with no symptoms, and as the CMV-infected lesions expanded, it was later recognized as CMVR [25–27]. Case 8 had the highest aqueous humor viral load, reaching 3.07×10^7 copies/mL, the blood CD4$^+$ lymphocyte count of the patient before relapse decreased from 253/mm^3 to 195/mm^3 within 2 months, and the patient received an intraocular dexamethasone intravitreal implant injection. These two factors suggest that while immune reconstitution is complete, intraocular hormone injection should be administered with caution under the protection of antiviral drugs, otherwise it could cause serious recurrence.

This article summarizes the characteristics of recurrent fundus lesions. The p-value of the correlation analysis between the initial visual acuity and lesion area at the time of recurrence was 0.064, suggesting that the wider the range of the recurrent lesions, the worse the visual prognosis was, especially when the lesions involved the optic disc and macula concurrently. In addition, CMVR recurrent lesions presented as yellow foci developing around the edge of the original focus, suggesting that the edge of the CMVR focus was the main site of inflammatory response between virus and tissue. Holland et al. also believed that the degree of opacity of the lesion margin was related to the immune status and prognosis of CMVR patients [28]. The higher the edge opacity of the lesion and the closer the lesion to the posterior pole, the greater the threat to vision, and the more active intraocular antiviral treatment was required [29].

In this study, the OCT images of the lesion area were analyzed and described. OCT can also show the changes in vitreous in the process of CMVR. The liquefaction and contraction of the vitreous body stimulated by the inflammation will stretch the necrotic lesions, forming tiny holes, which would eventually lead to retinal detachment. This study also observed one eye with tractional retinal detachment secondary to severe vitreoretinal proliferation, which differs slightly from a previous report that suggests that patients with CMVR have rhegmatogenous retinal detachment [30]. Risk factors for retinal detachment in CMVR include large areas of retinitis, bilateral involvement, and large areas of active lesions near the vitreous base [11]. Therefore, the application of OCT in clinical follow-ups is also of great significance for observing CMVR lesions. It can detect subtle changes in the vitreoretinal interface early and remind doctors to effectively intervene in high-risk patients to avoid serious complications.

By collecting and summarizing CMVR recurrence patient data after HSCT, this paper discusses the specificity of $CD4^{+}$ T cell count, viral load, fundus photography, and OCT characteristics from different perspectives. This study had a few limitations. The number of samples collected from patients is small because of population specificity, and the medication and treatment of this systemic disease cannot be unified. This caused difficulties in case collection, creating inevitable research bias, a problem that should be considered in similar studies going forward.

5. Conclusions

This study suggests that the clinical features, fundus manifestations, and imaging features of CMVR recurrence after HSCT are different from those at the initial onset. Patients should be closely followed up after their condition is stable to be alert to CMVR recurrence.

Author Contributions: Methodology, Y.L. and X.W.; software, X.W.; resources, J.H. and Z.M.; data curation, Y.L. and H.L.; writing—original draft preparation, X.W.; writing—review and editing, C.W. All authors have read and agreed to the published version of the manuscript.

Funding: National Natural Science Foundation: The process and mechanism of corneal endothelitis caused by cytomegalovirus infection (81970768).

Institutional Review Board Statement: This study was approved by the Ethics Committee of Peking University Third Hospital. Ethics approval number: 2015; Medical Ethics Review number: 197. The study followed the principles of the Declaration of Helsinki.

Informed Consent Statement: Informed consent was obtained from all subjects involved in the study.

Data Availability Statement: The clinical data in this study involve patient privacy and cannot be disclosed temporarily.

Conflicts of Interest: The authors declare no conflict of interest.

References

1. Zuhair, M.; Smit, G.; Wallis, G.; Jabbar, F.; Smith, C.; Devleesschauwer, B.; Griffiths, P. Estimation of the worldwide seroprevalence of cytomegalovirus: A systematic review and meta-analysis. *Rev. Med. Virol.* **2019**, *29*, e2034. [CrossRef]
2. Green, M.; Leisenring, W.; Xie, H.; Mast, T.; Cui, Y.; Sandmaier, B.; Sorror, M.; Goyal, S.; Özkök, S.; Yi, J.; et al. Cytomegalovirus viral load and mortality after haemopoietic stem cell transplantation in the era of pre-emptive therapy: A retrospective cohort study. *Lancet Haematol.* **2016**, *3*, e119–e127. [CrossRef]
3. Inamoto, Y.; Petriček, I.; Burns, L.; Chhabra, S.; DeFilipp, Z.; Hematti, P.; Rovó, A.; Schears, R.; Shah, A.; Agrawal, V.; et al. Non-GVHD ocular complications after hematopoietic cell transplantation: Expert review from the Late Effects and Quality of Life Working Committee of the CIBMTR and Transplant Complications Working Party of the EBMT. *Bone Marrow Transpl.* **2019**, *54*, 648–661. [CrossRef]
4. Vassallo, F.; Nuzzi, R.; Cattani, I.; Dellacasa, C.; Giaccone, L.; De Rosa, F.G.; Cavallo, R.; Iovino, G.; Brunello, L.; Bruno, B.; et al. CMV retinitis in a stem cell transplant recipient treated with foscarnet intravitreal injection and CMV specific immunoglobulins. *Ther. Adv. Hematol.* **2020**, *11*, 2040620720975651. [CrossRef]

5. Carmichael, A. Cytomegalovirus and the eye. *Eye* **2012**, *26*, 237–240. [CrossRef]
6. Mao, F.; Sun, H.; Li, D.; Wang, S.; Lu, D. Diagnostic analysis of Optos panoramic laser scanning ophthalmoscope and aqueous humor detection in patients with acquired immunodeficiency syndrome and cytomegalovirus retinitis. *Chin. J. Ocul. Fundus Dis.* **2021**, *37*, 509–512.
7. Pellegrini, M.; Bernabei, F.; Barbato, F.; Arpinati, M.; Giannaccare, G.; Versura, P.; Bonifazi, F. Incidence, risk factors and complications of ocular graft-versus-host disease following hematopoietic stem cell transplantation. *Am. J. Ophthalmol.* **2021**, *227*, 25–34. [CrossRef]
8. Long, Z.; Hou, J.; Miao, H. Neovascular complications from cytomegalovirus necrotizing retinopathy in patients after haploidentical hematopoietic stem cell transplantation. *Retina* **2021**, *41*, 1526–1532. [CrossRef]
9. Meng, X.; Fu, H.; Zhu, X.; Wang, J.; Liu, X.; Yan, C.; Zhang, Y.; Mo, X.; Wang, Y.; Han, W.; et al. Comparison of different cytomegalovirus diseases following haploidentical hematopoietic stem cell transplantation. *Ann. Hematol.* **2020**, *99*, 2659–2670. [CrossRef]
10. Holland, G.N.; Vaudaux, J.D.; Jeng, S.M.; Yu, F.; Goldenberg, D.T.; Folz, I.C.; Cumberland, W.G.; McCannel, C.A.; Helm, C.J.; Hardy, W.D. UCLA CMV Retinitis Study Group. Characteristics of untreated AIDS-related cytomegalovirus retinitis. I. Findings before the era of highly active antiretroviral therapy (1988 to 1994). *Am. J. Ophthalmol.* **2008**, *145*, 5–11. [CrossRef]
11. Port, A.D.; Orlin, A.; Kiss, S.; Patel, S.; D'Amico, D.J.; Gupta, M.P. Cytomegalovirus retinitis: A review. *J. Ocul. Pharmacol. Ther.* **2017**, *33*, 224–234. [CrossRef]
12. Lu, Y.; Hong, J.; Li, H.; Wang, X.; Ma, Z.; Wang, C. Relationship between opacity of cytomegalovirus retinitis lesion borders and aqueous viral load among patients after allogeneic hematopoietic stem cell transplantation. *Chin. J. Ophthalmol.* **2022**, *58*, 1033–1038.
13. Mo, W.; Chen, X.; Zhang, X.; Wang, S.; Li, L.; Zhang, Y. The Potential Association of Delayed T Lymphocyte Reconstitution Within Six Months Post-Transplantation With the Risk of Cytomegalovirus Retinitis in Severe Aplastic Anemia Recipients. *Front. Cell. Infect. Microbiol.* **2022**, *25*, 900154. [CrossRef]
14. Zhu, X.; Xiao, Y.; Zhang, W.; Lu, P. Detection of Intraocular Fluid and Infectious Diseases Study Clinical features of cytomegalovirus retinitis-associated uveitis in patients undergoing hematopoietic stem cell transplantation. *Chin. J. Ocul. Fundus Dis.* **2021**, *37*, 518–522.
15. AIDS Group, Society of Tropical Diseases and Parasitology of Zhejiang Medical Association. Zhejiang expert consensus on diagnosis and treatment of cytomegalovirus retinitis in AIDS patients. *Chin. J. Clin. Infect. Dis.* **2019**, *12*, 331–338.
16. Zhang, J.; Kamoi, K.; Zong, Y.; Yang, M.; Ohno-Matsui, K. Cytomegalovirus Anterior Uveitis: Clinical Manifestations, Diagnosis, Treatment, and Immunological Mechanisms. *Viruses* **2023**, *15*, 185. [CrossRef]
17. Yu, Y.Y.; Zhao, M.W.; Miao, H. Regime for cytomegalovirus retinitis based on aqueous virology and inflammatory cytokine determination. *Chin. J. Ocul. Fundus Dis.* **2020**, *36*, 1–4.
18. Atay, D.; Akcay, A.; Erbey, F.; Ozturk, G. The impact of alternative donor types on viral infections in pediatric hematopoietic stem cell transplantation. *Pediatr. Transpl.* **2018**, *22*, e13109. [CrossRef]
19. Chan, S.T.; Logan, A.C. The clinical impact of cytomegalovirus infection following allogeneic hematopoietic cell transplantation: Why the quest for meaningful prophylaxis still matters. *Blood Rev.* **2017**, *31*, 173–183. [CrossRef]
20. Bhatt, S.; Bednarski, J. Immune Reconstitution in Pediatric Patients Following Hematopoietic Cell Transplant for Non-malignant Disorders. *Front. Immunol.* **2020**, *18*, 1988. [CrossRef]
21. Iu, L.P.; Fan, M.C.; Lau, J.K.; Chan, T.S.; Kwong, Y.L.; Wong, I.Y. Long-term follow-up of cytomegalovirus retinitis in non-HIV immunocompromised patients: Clinical features and visual prognosis. *Am. J. Ophthalmol.* **2016**, *165*, 145–153. [CrossRef]
22. Kim, J.; Hong, S.; Park, W.; Kim, R.; Kim, M.; Park, Y.; Kim, H.; Lee, S.; Lee, D.; Park, Y. Prognostic factors of cytomegalovirus retinitis after hematopoietic stem cell transplantation. *PLoS ONE* **2020**, *15*, e0238257. [CrossRef]
23. Jeon, S.; Lee, W.; Lee, Y.; Lee, D.; Lee, J. Risk factors for cytomegalovirus retinitis in patients with cytomegalovirus viremia after hematopoietic stem cell transplantation. *Ophthalmology* **2012**, *119*, 1892–1898. [CrossRef]
24. Chen, W.; Long, Z.; Hou, J.; Miao, H.; Zhao, M. Continuous High-Dose (6 mg) vs. Low-Dose (3 mg) Intravitreal Ganciclovir for Cytomegalovirus Retinitis After Haploidentical Hematopoietic Stem Cell Transplantation: A Randomized Controlled Study. *Front. Med.* **2021**, *24*, 750760. [CrossRef]
25. Suzuki, K.; Namba, K.; Mizuuchi, K.; Iwata, D.; Ito, T.; Hase, K.; Kitaichi, N.; Ishida, S. Development of cytomegalovirus retinitis after negative conversion of cytomegalovirus antigenemia due to systemic antiviral therapy. *Graefe's Arch. Clin. Exp. Ophthalmol.* **2021**, *259*, 971–978. [CrossRef]
26. Shapira, Y.; Mimouni, M.; Vishnevskia-Dai, V. Cytomegalovirus retinitis in HIV-negative patients-associated conditions, clinical presentation, diagnostic methods and treatment strategy. *Acta Ophthalmol.* **2018**, *96*, e761–e767. [CrossRef]
27. Hong, S.; Kim, T.; Park, S.; Jung, J.; Lee, J.; Chong, Y.; Sung, H.; Lee, S.; Choi, S.; Kim, Y.; et al. Sensitivity of the Cytomegalovirus Antigenemia Assay to Diagnose Cytomegalovirus Retinitis. *Infect. Chemother.* **2016**, *48*, 302–308. [CrossRef]
28. Holland, G.N.; Van Natta, M.L.; Goldenberg, D.T.; Ritts, R., Jr.; Danis, R.P.; Jabs, D.A.; Studies of Ocular Complications of AIDS Research Group. Relationship between opacity of cytomegalovirus retinitis lesion borders and severity of immunodeficiency among people with AIDS. *Investig. Ophthalmol. Vis. Sci.* **2019**, *60*, 1853–1862. [CrossRef]

29. Heng, M.; Jing, H. Influent factors for treating procedure of cytomegalovirus retinitis after allogeneic bone marrow hematopoietic stem cell transplantation. *Chin. J. Ophthalmol.* **2017**, *53*, 740–745.
30. Fan, J.J.; Tao, Y.; Hwang, D.K. Comparison of intravitreal ganciclovir monotherapy and combination with foscarnet as initial therapy for cytomegalovirus retinitis. *Int. J. Ophthalmol.* **2018**, *11*, 1638–1642.

Journal of *Personalized Medicine*

MDPI

Article

Automatic Diagnosis of Infectious Keratitis Based on Slit Lamp Images Analysis

Shaodan Hu [1,†], Yiming Sun [1,†], Jinhao Li [2], Peifang Xu [1], Mingyu Xu [1], Yifan Zhou [1], Yaqi Wang [3], Shuai Wang [2,4,*] and Juan Ye [1,*]

1 Department of Ophthalmology, College of Medicine, The Second Affiliated Hospital of Zhejiang University, Hangzhou 310009, China
2 School of Mechanical, Electrical and Information Engineering, Shandong University, Weihai 264209, China
3 College of Media Engineering, Communication University of Zhejiang, Hangzhou 310018, China; wangyaqi@cuz.edu.cn
4 Suzhou Research Institute, Shandong University, Suzhou 215123, China
* Correspondence: shuaiwang.tai@gmail.com (S.W.); yejuan@zju.edu.cn (J.Y.)
† These authors contributed equally to this work.

Abstract: Infectious keratitis (IK) is a common ophthalmic emergency that requires prompt and accurate treatment. This study aimed to propose a deep learning (DL) system based on slit lamp images to automatically screen and diagnose infectious keratitis. This study established a dataset of 2757 slit lamp images from 744 patients, including normal cornea, viral keratitis (VK), fungal keratitis (FK), and bacterial keratitis (BK). Six different DL algorithms were developed and evaluated for the classification of infectious keratitis. Among all the models, the EffecientNetV2-M showed the best classification ability, with an accuracy of 0.735, a recall of 0.680, and a specificity of 0.904, which was also superior to two ophthalmologists. The area under the receiver operating characteristics curve (AUC) of the EffecientNetV2-M was 0.85; correspondingly, 1.00 for normal cornea, 0.87 for VK, 0.87 for FK, and 0.64 for BK. The findings suggested that the proposed DL system could perform well in the classification of normal corneas and different types of infectious keratitis, based on slit lamp images. This study proves the potential of the DL model to help ophthalmologists to identify infectious keratitis and improve the accuracy and efficiency of diagnosis.

Keywords: deep learning; infectious keratitis; slit lamp image; automatic classification

Citation: Hu, S.; Sun, Y.; Li, J.; Xu, P.; Xu, M.; Zhou, Y.; Wang, Y.; Wang, S.; Ye, J. Automatic Diagnosis of Infectious Keratitis Based on Slit Lamp Images Analysis. *J. Pers. Med.* **2023**, *13*, 519. https://doi.org/10.3390/jpm13030519

Academic Editor: Yousif Subhi

Received: 11 February 2023
Revised: 5 March 2023
Accepted: 9 March 2023
Published: 13 March 2023

1. Introduction

Corneal opacity is the fifth-leading cause of blindness worldwide [1], and infectious keratitis (IK) is the leading cause of corneal blindness in both developed and developing countries [2]. The most prominent feature of IK is that the growth of pathogens in the cornea leads to local opacity and roughness, and each pathogen shows its unique characteristics in the growth [3]. According to the types of pathogens, infectious keratitis can be divided into bacterial keratitis (BK) [4], fungal keratitis (FK) [5], and viral keratitis (VK) [6]. Once corneal infection occurs, it may progress rapidly, leading to irreversible visual impairments such as corneal scars, endophthalmitis, and corneal perforation [7]. Therefore, early detection and timely medical intervention are critical to stop or slow the progression of the infection.

Corneal scrape culture is currently the gold standard for the diagnosis of IK, but there are drawbacks, such as the risk of corneal injury, the low positive rate of culture, and long diagnostic cycles [8,9]. New techniques such as polymerase chain reaction (PCR) [10–12] and confocal microscopy [13] have also been used clinically to assist in diagnosis, but these methods require sophisticated equipment, complex procedures and experienced technicians. At present, the initial diagnosis of IK is highly dependent on ophthalmologists, who need to combine personal experience to distinguish the visual features of corneal lesions. Slit lamp microscopy is the most common ophthalmologic examination used to evaluate the appearance of IK. Slit lamp photographs are commonly used to record and monitor the progression of IK [14]. However, because of the diversity of pathogens and the similarity of lesion manifestations, it is difficult to identify different IK, even for experienced corneal specialists. Overall, there is still a lack of an efficient and accurate diagnostic tool to help guide the treatment of infectious keratitis in clinical practice.

In recent years, artificial intelligence (AI) technology has developed rapidly, and medicine has become the frontier area of AI applications. Recent studies of deep learning (DL) have shown great promise in the use of clinical images to detect common diseases [15]. The convolutional neural network (CNN), as its representative algorithm, has been proven to be very effective in medical image recognition and classification [16]. The automatic classification of medical images can not only reduce the workload of doctors and improve the efficiency and repeatability of screening procedures, but also improve patient outcomes through early detection and treatment. Although there are more than 200,000 ophthalmologists worldwide, there is a current and anticipated future shortage in the number of ophthalmologists in both developing and developed countries [17]. The widening gap between demand and supply can affect the timely detection of infectious keratitis, especially in remote or medically underserved areas [18]. In situations where ophthalmologists are in short supply or medical resources are limited, artificial intelligence is expected to become a practical tool for front-line medical care.

In the field of ophthalmology, a large number of studies have developed high-precision AI diagnostic systems based on rich examinations and image data for diseases of the posterior segment of the eye, such as diabetic retinopathy, glaucomatous optic neuropathy, and retinal detachment [19–21]. The application progress of deep learning in different fundus diseases has extended to early screening, grading and stage diagnosis and even to the prediction of treatment effects [22–24]. In contrast, the application of deep learning in anterior segment diseases is limited and has great research potential. Recent studies have attempted to apply deep learning to slit lamp images for the diagnosis of corneal diseases. Gu et al. [25] developed a DL model to identify infectious keratitis, non-infectious keratitis, corneal dystrophy or degeneration, and corneal neoplasm, with results similar to their ophthalmologists. However, to our knowledge, the application of DL to the classification of pathogens in infectious keratitis remains limited.

Thus, we decided to construct a deep learning system for the automatic classification of slit lamp images to achieve an intelligent diagnosis of infectious keratitis, which could offer assistance to ophthalmologists in screening and diagnosing infectious keratitis. We hope that it will help reduce the rate of clinical misdiagnoses, save patients' vision, and further alleviate the burden on medical resources and society's economy.

2. Methods

2.1. Image Dataset

This study retrospectively established a dataset that included 2757 slit lamp images collected from 744 patients between August 2016 and September 2021 in the Eye Center at the Second Affiliated Hospital of the Zhejiang University School of Medicine. The images were acquired by experienced ophthalmic technicians using two Topcon SL-D701 slit lamp biomicroscopes affixed with DC-4 digital cameras in the diffuse illumination mode. In the slit lamp image dataset, 2165 images were taken from IK patients at the active stage, including bacterial keratitis (BK), fungal keratitis (FK) and viral keratitis (VK). In addition, 592 images taken from healthy eyes with negative fluorescence staining were classified into the category of normal cornea. The representative images for each category are shown in Figure 1.

All cases of IK were diagnosed by cornea specialists from our center, based on medical histories, clinical manifestations, corneal examinations, laboratory methods, and follow-up outcomes. The diagnostic labels based on the medical records' information were considered to be the true labels of this study. The diagnostic criteria were (1) BK: positive corneal scraping results for bacteria (microscopic staining or tissue culture); (2) FK: positive corneal scraping results for fungi (microscopic staining or tissue culture) or fungal hyphae found under confocal microscopy; (3) VK: positive PCR test results for viruses on corneal scraping; (4) the corresponding typical clinical history; (5) the corresponding typical manifestations of corneal lesions; (6) the corresponding anti-pathogenic drugs were effective. The first three are laboratory gold standards, wherein one of which must be met; the last three are auxiliary indicators, at least one of which must be met. The exclusion criteria were (1) patients with not enough evidence for a definite diagnosis or with mixed infections; (2) patients with corneal perforation, corneal scarring, a history of corneal surgery, or other corneal diseases; (3) images with poor quality, including poor-field, defocused, and poor-location images. Images that met any of the above criteria were excluded. Our two researchers independently reviewed all data in detail before any analysis and ensured that each image was correctly matched to the specific individual.

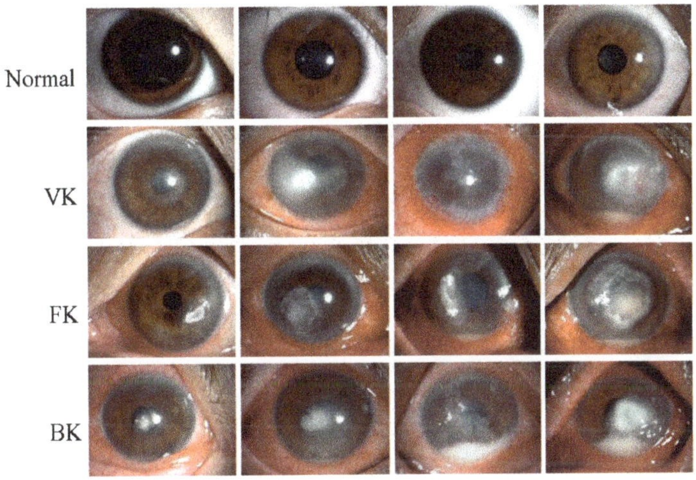

Figure 1. Representative slit lamp images of the normal cornea (Normal), viral keratitis (VK), fungal keratitis (FK), and bacterial keratitis (BK), from top to bottom. Each image was from a different eye, and each category of keratitis showed a different degree of infection.

2.2. Data Preparation

The slit lamp images were initially preprocessed, including with shuffle and normalization. For each category of images, the dataset was divided into a training set, validation set and test set. For reducing the impact of the dataset imbalance, the ratio of the BK was adjusted to 0.65:0.2:0.15 and the other three groups were 7:1:2. All images collected from the same patient were only divided into the same dataset to avoid data information leakage from the test set and incorrect evaluation of the model performance. The distribution of the slit lamp image datasets is shown in Table 1.

Data augmentation is an essential approach to automatically generate new training samples and improve the generalization of the DL models [26]. We obtained samples using several strategies: (1) random cropping images with ranges of (0%, 30%); (2) random rotation with ranges of (−10°, +10°); (3) color jitter with ranges of (−10%, + 10%); (4) random horizontal flip; (5) adding Gaussian noise with mean = 0, variance = 1, and amplitude = 8. In addition, we tripled the sample size of the BK to reduce the effect of dataset imbalance. Finally, each image was resized to 224 × 224 pixels to be compatible with the original dimensions of the experiment networks.

Table 1. The distribution of the slit lamp image datasets.

Dataset (*n*)	Normal	VK	FK	BK	Total
Training	425	583	753	164	1925
Validation	60	79	127	35	301
Test	107	151	245	28	531
Total	592	813	1125	227	2757

2.3. Deep Learning Model

Figure 2A shows the flowchart of the DL system for the automatic diagnosis of IK based on slit lamp images. For the development of the DL diagnosis models, we applied various classical and efficient algorithms, including VGG16 [27], ResNet34 [28], InceptionV4 [29], DenseNet121 [30], ViT-Base [31] and EffecientNetV2-M [32]. The above networks are all CNN structures, except for ViT, which uses the Transformer structure. As the latest algorithm proposed in 2021, EffecientNetV2 has achieved state-of-the-art performance in many major image classification tasks, and its structure is shown in Figure 2B.

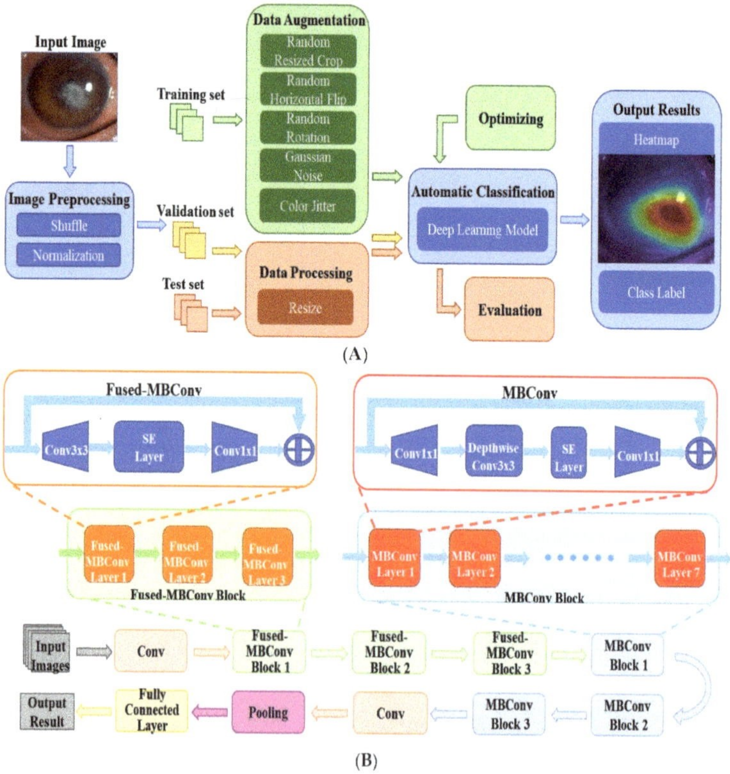

Figure 2. (**A**) The flowchart of the DL diagnostic system for IK based on slit lamp images. Firstly, the input images were preprocessed and divided into three data sets. Next, data augmentation and data processing were performed on the images. Then, various DL algorithms were used for model development, optimization, and evaluation. Finally, the results of the models were output in the form of heatmaps and class labels. (**B**) The architecture of EfficientNetV2. It was mainly composed of several Fused-MBConv blocks and MBConv blocks. Early features were extracted using Fused-MBConv blocks, which used 1×1 Conv, 3×3 Conv and SE layers. It used depthwise convolution to extract from MBConv blocks. Compared with the traditional convolution widely used in other models, depthwise convolution had fewer parameters and computation.

The training set was used to train the DL models for differentiating infectious keratitis, whereas the validation set was used to verify their performance. All models were implemented using the Pytorch platform with an Nvidia RTX 2080TI GPU. For each model, 150 epochs were set for the training, and the batch size was set at 15. During model training, RMSPromp optimizer and cosine annealing were applied to help the model converge quickly. Moreover, hyperparameter tuning was used to optimize all models according to the validation results. The test set was used to evaluate the performance of the optimal model. The heatmaps were plotted by the Gradient-weighted Class Activation Mapping (Grad-CAM) technique [33]. It can generate visual interpretations for CNN-based deep learning models to build trust in the predicted results and provide references for doctors.

2.4. Performance Assessment

Six different DL models in this study were evaluated in an independent test set, and the images obtained from the same patient were not scattered to different datasets. The performance of the DL models for the classification of IK was evaluated by calculating the accuracy, recall and specificity. Statistical analyses were conducted using Python 3.8.10 (Wilmington, DE, USA) and Pycharm 2021.1.3 (Professional edition). To compare the classification ability of the models, the receiver operating characteristics (ROC) curves were created using the packages Scikit-learn (version 0.24.2) and Matplotlib (version 3.2.2). The horizontal axis of the ROC curve is the false positive rate (FPR), which is 1-specificity, and the vertical axis is the true positive rate (TPR), which is the recall. The area under the ROC curve (AUC) can measure classification performance. The closer the value of AUC is to 1, the better the performance is. We also recruited two ophthalmologists to independently classify the same test set and evaluate their classification results using the same metrics. Then, the classification performance of the best-performing model was compared by two ophthalmologists (i.e., Doctor 1 and Doctor 2). The confusion matrices were plotted by Matplotlib (version 3.2.2), which is helpful in analyzing the misclassification of each category by the model and ophthalmologists.

3. Results

3.1. Performance of the DL Models

Six DL algorithms were used in this study to train the models for the classification of BK, VK, FK and normal cornea. The performance of these DL models in the test set was evaluated by accuracy, recall, and specificity, as shown in Table 2. The best classification algorithm was EffecientNetV2-M, with an accuracy of 0.735, a recall of 0.680, and a specificity of 0.904. Doctor 1 and Doctor 2 reached an accuracy of 0.661 and 0.685, a recall of 0.636 and 0.648, and a specificity of 0.884 and 0.891, respectively.

Table 2. Performance comparison of six DL models for IK classification.

Model	Accuracy	Recall	Specificity
ResNet34	0.635	0.554	0.861
DenseNet121	0.637	0.637	0.875
ViT-Base	0.697	0.598	0.888
VGG16	0.708	0.583	0.890
InceptionV4	0.716	0.640	0.897
EffecientNetV2-M	0.735	0.680	0.904

The macro-average ROC curves of the six DL models are shown in Figure 3. InceptionV4 reached the highest AUC value of 0.86, while EffectNetV2-M reached 0.85, higher than other models (VGG16 AUC = 0.83, ResNet34 AUC = 0.82, ViT-Base AUC = 0.82, DenseNet121 AUC = 0.81).

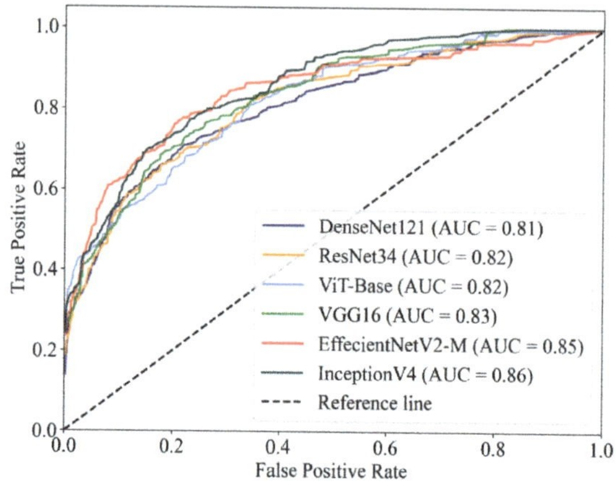

Figure 3. The macro-average ROC curves and AUCs of six DL models. The AUCs of the models ranged from 0.81–0.86.

3.2. Comparison with the Ophthalmologists

Figure 4A compares the macro-average ROC curves between the EffecientNetV2-M model and the ophthalmologists. The EffecientNetV2-M model achieved an AUC of 0.85, higher than two ophthalmologists, which were 0.76 and 0.77, respectively. The ROC curves of the EffecientNetV2-M model for each category are shown in Figure 4B, with Doctor 1 corresponding to Figure 4C and Doctor 2 corresponding to Figure 4D. For the AUCs of each category, the EffecientNetV2-M model, Doctor 1 and Doctor 2 reached a normal cornea AUC of 1.00, 0.89 and 0.97, respectively; VK of 0.87, 0.75 and 0.78, respectively; FK of 0.87, 0.74 and 0.72, respectively; and BK of 0.64, 0.66 and 0.61, respectively.

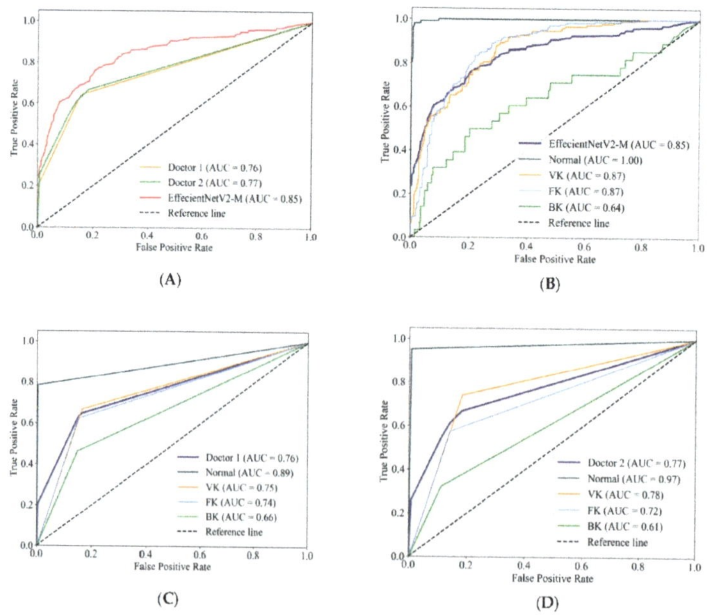

Figure 4. The macro-average ROC curves and AUCs of the EffecientNetV2-M model and two ophthalmologists (**A**). The ROC curves for each category of the EffecientNetV2-M model (**B**), Doctor 1 (**C**) and Doctor 2 (**D**).

Figure 5A,B shows the confusion matrices of the EffecientNetV2-M model and the average results of the two ophthalmologists. The horizontal axis represents the true category labels, and the vertical axis represents the predicted category labels. As the green color of the matrix deepens, it means that the value increases. The distribution of the last line shows the difficulty of classifying BK, where the real BK is easily misjudged as FK, either by the DL model or by the ophthalmologists. In addition, it can be seen that the model is more likely to recognize the real VK as the other groups, whereas the ophthalmologist is more likely to recognize the other groups as VK. The confusion matrix reveals the similarities and differences between the algorithm and the ophthalmologists in misclassification.

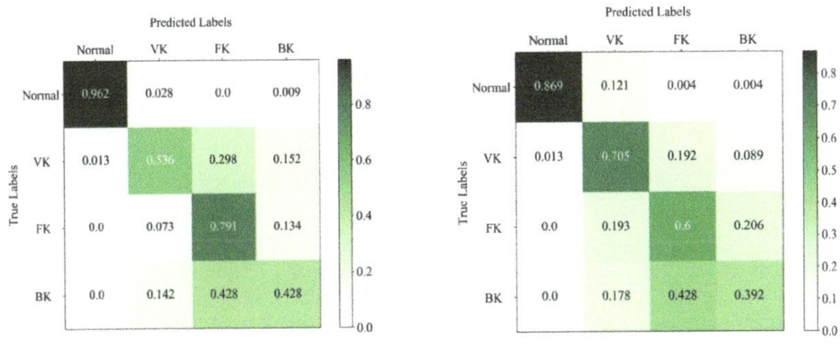

(A) (B)

Figure 5. The confusion matrix of the EffecientNetV2-M model (**A**) and the average results of two ophthalmologists (**B**) in the test set. The column denotes the predicted labels, and the row indicates the true labels.

3.3. Heatmaps

Figure 6 presents examples of heatmaps generated by the EffecientNetV2-M model, accompanied by the corresponding original image. The redder regions represent the areas that are of greater concern during the model classification process, and the bluer regions represent those of relatively less concern. The heatmaps highlighted the areas with corneal lesions, which are highly correlated with the identification of infectious keratitis.

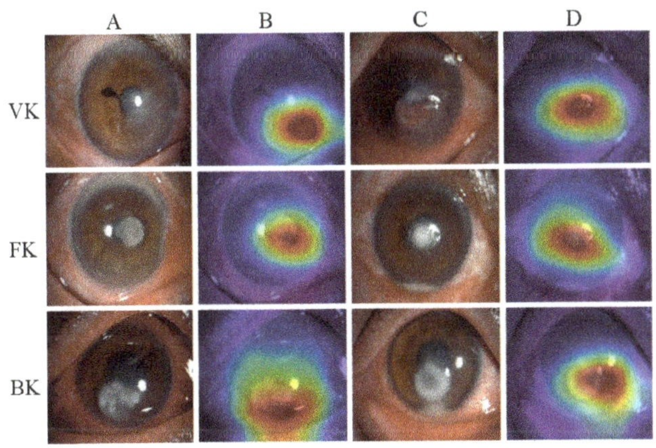

Figure 6. The heatmaps generated by the EffecientNetV2-M model. From top to bottom, each row corresponds to the images of viral keratitis (VK), fungal keratitis (FK) and bacterial keratitis (BK). Columns (**A**,**C**) are different original image examples of images of each category, while column (**B**) are the heatmaps generated by column (**A**), and column (**D**) are the heatmaps generated by column (**C**).

3.4. Discussion

As a common emergency in ophthalmology, timely and accurate treatment is essential for the prognosis of infectious keratitis. However, the diagnosis of infectious keratitis is a huge challenge clinically due to the diversity of pathogens and the similarity of clinical manifestations. In this study, we constructed a DL diagnosis system for IK to automatically classify BK, FK, VK, and normal corneas by analyzing slit lamp images. Six DL models were developed using the same dataset and compared with the performance of two ophthalmologists. In the end, the EffecientNetV2-M model performed better than the other models and the ophthalmologists, with an accuracy of 0.735, a recall of 0.680, and a specificity of 0.904. Our results suggested that the DL model could be useful for ophthalmologists to screen and diagnose infectious keratitis, thereby reducing the rate of misdiagnosis clinically, saving patients' vision, and further alleviating the burden of medical resources and socioeconomic issues. In addition, DL technology makes it possible to provide telemedicine services for the diagnosis of IK in places where timely ophthalmologic assessment cannot be performed, such as in rural areas.

Recently, some studies have attempted to apply deep learning to slit lamp images for the diagnosis of keratitis. Kuo et al. [34] identified fungal and nonfungal keratitis using the DenseNet network based on 288 corneal photographs, with an accuracy of 69.4% and an AUC of 0.65. Ghosh et al. [35] adopted the ensemble technique for identifying BK and FK based on 194 cases, obtaining a recall rate of 0.77 and an F1 score of 0.83. Li et al. [36] developed a DL system that can automatically classify keratitis, other cornea abnormalities, and normal corneas with slit lamp and smartphone images, with an AUC of more than 0.96. Xu et al. [37] compared three image-level algorithms for the classification of BK, FK, HSK, and other corneal disorders, with the DenseNet model achieving optimal accuracy (64.17%), which was superior to 421 ophthalmologists (49.27 ± 11.5%). In addition, a large international study [38] quantified the performance of 66 cornea specialists in the image-based differentiation of BK and FK, with AUCs of 0.39–0.82 (mean of 0.61).

Compared with the previous studies, the advantages of this study are as follows. First, we collected and built a relatively large and diverse image dataset, including 2757 slit lamp images from 744 patients. Furthermore, the classification task of this study was relatively more complex—to distinguish BK, FK, VK, and normal cornea. Next, we evaluated and compared the classification performance of six different models and two ophthalmologists. The EffecientNetV2 model outperformed other classical models and ophthalmologists in this study, achieving an AUC of 0.85 and an accuracy of 0.735. The ophthalmologists reached an AUC of 0.76 and 0.77, with an accuracy of 0.661 and 0.685, respectively. Our results were better than most previous studies. It is significant that the EffecientNetV2 algorithm used in this study is currently the latest and strongest CNN, which improves the index by comprehensively optimizing the network width, network depth and resolution. Lastly, visual heatmaps were generated to make our DL system interpretable. The heatmaps of the EffecientNetV2-M model highlighted areas that were highly correlated with the lesions of IK. The interpretability of this model can be useful in real-world applications, as it can help ophthalmologists understand how the DL system produces the final output.

The EffecientNetV2-M model performed best in this study, but its ability to classify different types of IK varied. The AUCs of the normal cornea, VK, FK and BK were 1.00, 0.87, 0.87 and 0.64, respectively. This means that the model has a strong classification ability to distinguish normal cornea images from infectious keratitis and has a good classification effect for VK and FK, but not so good for BK. The possible reasons are as follows: (1) each species of BK may have different lesion characteristics, and the same species may even have different manifestations in different stages of infection, which makes the classification difficult; (2) different types of IK (especially BK and FK) may have similar lesion characteristics, which may lead to their misclassification; (3) the number of images in each group is relatively limited (especially BK), which leads to the failure of the DL models to learn the unique features of various types of keratitis comprehensively. According to the confusion matrices, about half of the real BK images were misjudged as FK by both the DL algorithm and the ophthalmologists. This confirmed that the lesion characteristics of BK and FK are similar, which makes visual diagnosis challenging. In addition, comparing the misclassification between the algorithm and the ophthalmologists may help improve the diagnostic model. However, it must be noted that few clinicians use only a single slit lamp image to diagnose infectious keratitis. The optical quality of the image may affect their judgment, such as in the presence of reflection and artifacts. Therefore, these factors may lead to inconsistency and error when ophthalmologists perform this classification task.

There are also some limitations in this study. First, the dataset was still relatively inadequate compared with some large studies, and cases were not well balanced across groups. In particular, the number of BK images is relatively small, which may also be the main reason for the poor classification effect of BK. The relatively limited number of BK patients may be due to the empirical clinical use of antibiotic eye drops, resulting in a low probability of the laboratory detection of the bacteria. In contrast, bacteria with stronger antibiotic resistance are easier to be detected but are usually accompanied by serious clinical manifestations such as hypopyon. Fortunately, recent studies may have found effective treatments for drug-resistant bacterial corneal infection [39,40]. For us, an early collection of untreated keratitis images may be a solution to increasing the number of BK images. Second, we only evaluated the performance of the developed model on an internal dataset. Various data enhancement processes were used to increase the diversity of the datasets to prevent overfitting and improve the reliability of the training model. However, it is currently difficult to conclude whether the model can be used to screen real patients. In the future, we will collect more cases for model development and validation, including data from multiple centers. Third, we excluded mixed infections with different types of keratitis in this study, although this condition is very common clinically. We believe that identifying mixed infections is a much larger and more difficult deep-learning task. The DL models must fully learn the characterization of each keratitis before it is possible to identify two or more types of keratitis infections. This may require a good understanding of the unique lesion characteristics of different IK, such as corneal infiltration, bacterial or fungal moss, hypopyon and so on. By combining the manual labeling of corneal lesions, it may be possible to improve the focus of the model on the lesion and learn more comprehensive information. In addition, the combination of the model with relevant clinical history information (e.g., trauma, underlying disease, medication history, etc.) may also be a method to enhance model recognition ability. Lastly, our model could not identify the degree or stage of the keratitis infection. We believe that this recognition task needs corneal multi-level information, and we are working on this by combining other corneal examinations, such as fluorescent staining, anterior segment optical coherence tomography (AS-OCT), corneal topography and so on. In any case, we believe that the DL diagnostic system can be further improved to better assist the identification of IK, which can help improve diagnostic accuracy and efficiency.

4. Conclusions

In this study, we proposed an intelligent diagnosis system for IK using DL technology to analyze slit lamp images. Compared with the other models and ophthalmologists, the EffecientNetV2-M model achieved higher accuracy and AUC in this study. The findings suggest that the proposed DL system could perform well in the classification of normal corneas and different types of infectious keratitis based on slit lamp images. This demonstrates the potential of the DL model to help ophthalmologists identify infectious keratitis, and it provides the possibility of improving diagnostic accuracy and efficiency.

Author Contributions: Conceptualization, S.H., Y.S., P.X. and J.Y.; methodology, J.L., Y.W. and S.W.; software, J.L.; validation, Y.S., M.X. and Y.Z.; formal analysis, S.H. and J.L.; investigation, S.H., M.X. and Y.Z.; resources, S.W. and J.Y.; data curation, S.H., Y.S. and P.X.; writing—original draft preparation, S.H., Y.S. and P.X.; writing—review and editing, Y.W., S.W. and J.Y.; visualization, J.L.; supervision, Y.W., S.W. and J.Y.; project administration, S.W. and J.Y.; funding acquisition, S.W. and J.Y. All authors have read and agreed to the published version of the manuscript.

Funding: This research was funded by the National Natural Science Foundation Regional Innovation and Development Joint Fund, grant number U20A20386, the National Natural Science Foundation of China, grant number 81870635, the Clinical Medical Research Center for Eye Diseases of Zhejiang Province, grant number 2021E50007, the National Natural Science Foundation of China, grant number 62201323, and the Natural Science Foundation of Jiangsu Province, grant number BK20220266.

Institutional Review Board Statement: The study was conducted in accordance with the Declaration of Helsinki and approved by the Ethics Committee of The Second Affiliated Hospital of Zhejiang University, School of Medicine (protocol code:2021-0263 and date of approval: 6 May 2021).

Informed Consent Statement: Patient consent was waived due to the retrospective nature of this study, in which identification information in slit lamp images was removed from all participants.

Data Availability Statement: The data are not publicly available due to privacy issues. Requests to access the datasets should be directed to the Second Affiliated Hospital of Zhejiang University, School of Medicine.

Conflicts of Interest: The authors declare no conflict of interest.

References

1. Flaxman, S.R.; Bourne, R.R.A.; Resnikoff, S.; Ackland, P.; Braithwaite, T.; Cicinelli, M.V.; Das, A.; Jonas, J.B.; Keeffe, J.; Kempen, J.H.; et al. Global causes of blindness and distance vision impairment 1990–2020: A systematic review and meta-analysis. *Lancet Glob. Health* **2017**, *5*, E1221–E1234. [CrossRef] [PubMed]
2. Ung, L.; Bispo, P.J.M.; Shanbhag, S.S.; Gilmore, M.S.; Chodosh, J. The persistent dilemma of microbial keratitis: Global burden, diagnosis and antimicrobial resistance. *Surv. Ophthalmol.* **2019**, *64*, 255–271. [CrossRef] [PubMed]
3. Gopinathan, U.; Garg, P.; Fernandes, M.; Sharma, S.; Athmanathan, S.; Rao, G.N. The epidemiological features and laboratory results of fungal keratitis: A 10-year review at a referral eye care center in South India. *Cornea* **2002**, *21*, 555–559. [CrossRef] [PubMed]
4. Clemens, L.E.; Jaynes, J.; Lim, E.; Kolar, S.S.; Reins, R.Y.; Baidouri, H.; Hanlon, S.; McDermott, A.M.; Woodburn, K.W. Designed Host Defense Peptides for the Treatment of Bacterial Keratitis. *Investig. Ophthalmol. Vis. Sci.* **2017**, *58*, 6273–6281. [CrossRef]
5. Leck, A.; Burton, M. Distinguishing fungal and bacterial keratitis on clinical signs. *Community Eye Health* **2015**, *28*, 6–7.
6. Mader, T.H.; Stulting, R.D. Viral keratitis. *Infect. Dis. Clin. N. Am.* **1992**, *6*, 831–849. [CrossRef]
7. Watson, S.; Cabrera-Aguas, M.; Khoo, P. Common eye infections. *Aust. Prescr.* **2018**, *41*, 67–72. [CrossRef]
8. Green, M.; Apel, A.; Stapleton, F. Risk factors and causative organisms in microbial keratitis. *Cornea* **2008**, *27*, 22–27. [CrossRef]
9. Shalchi, Z.; Gurbaxani, A.; Baker, M.; Nash, J. Antibiotic Resistance in Microbial Keratitis: Ten-Year Experience of Corneal Scrapes in the United Kingdom. *Ophthalmology* **2011**, *118*, 2161–2165. [CrossRef]
10. Brunner, M.; Somerville, T.; Corless, C.E.; Myneni, J.; Rajhbeharrysingh, T.; Tiew, S.; Neal, T.; Kaye, S.B. Use of a corneal impression membrane and PCR for the detection of herpes simplex virus type-1. *J. Med. Microbiol.* **2019**, *68*, 1324–1329. [CrossRef]
11. Geetha, D.K.; Sivaraman, B.; Rammohan, R.; Venkatapathy, N.; Ramatchandirane, P.S. A SYBR Green based multiplex Real-Time PCR assay for rapid detection and differentiation of ocular bacterial pathogens. *J. Microbiol. Methods* **2020**, *171*, 105875. [CrossRef]
12. Kulandai, L.T.; Lakshmipathy, D.; Sargunam, J. Novel Duplex Polymerase Chain Reaction for the Rapid Detection of Pythium insidiosum Directly from Corneal Specimens of Patients with Ocular Pythiosis. *Cornea* **2020**, *39*, 775–778. [CrossRef]
13. Wang, Y.E.; Tepelus, T.C.; Vickers, L.A.; Baghdasaryan, E.; Gui, W.; Huang, P.; Irvine, J.A.; Sadda, S.; Hsu, H.Y.; Lee, O.L. Role of in vivo confocal microscopy in the diagnosis of infectious keratitis. *Int. Ophthalmol.* **2019**, *39*, 2865–2874. [CrossRef]
14. Dalmon, C.; Porco, T.C.; Lietman, T.M.; Prajna, N.V.; Prajna, L.; Das, M.R.; Kumar, J.A.; Mascarenhas, J.; Margolis, T.P.; Whitcher, J.P.; et al. The Clinical Differentiation of Bacterial and Fungal Keratitis: A Photographic Survey. *Investig. Ophthalmol. Vis. Sci.* **2012**, *53*, 1787–1791. [CrossRef]
15. Chan, H.P.; Samala, R.K.; Hadjiiski, L.M.; Zhou, C. Deep Learning in Medical Image Analysis. In *Deep Learning in Medical Image Analysis: Challenges and Applications. Advances in Experimental Medicine and Biology*; Lee, G., Fujita, H., Eds.; IEEE: New York, NY, USA, 2020; Volume 1213, pp. 3–21.
16. Marques, G.; Agarwal, D.; de la Torre Díez, I. Automated medical diagnosis of COVID-19 through EfficientNet convolutional neural network. *Appl. Soft. Comput.* **2020**, *96*, 106691. [CrossRef]
17. Resnikoff, S.; Felch, W.; Gauthier, T.M.; Spivey, B. The number of ophthalmologists in practice and training worldwide: A growing gap despite more than 200,000 practitioners. *Br. J. Ophthalmol.* **2012**, *96*, 783–787. [CrossRef]
18. Gupta, N.; Tandon, R.; Gupta, S.K.; Sreenivas, V.; Vashist, P. Burden of corneal blindness in India. *Indian J. Commun. Med.* **2013**, *38*, 198–206.
19. Ting, D.S.W.; Cheung, C.Y.L.; Lim, G.; Tan, G.S.W.; Quang, N.D.; Gan, A.; Hamzah, H.; Garcia-Franco, R.; Yeo, I.Y.S.; Lee, S.Y.; et al. Development and Validation of a Deep Learning System for Diabetic Retinopathy and Related Eye Diseases Using Retinal Images from Multiethnic Populations with Diabetes. *J. Am. Med. Assoc.* **2017**, *318*, 2211–2223. [CrossRef]
20. Hood, D.C.; De Moraes, C.G. Efficacy of a Deep Learning System for Detecting Glaucomatous Optic Neuropathy Based on Color Fundus Photographs. *Ophthalmology* **2018**, *125*, 1207–1208. [CrossRef]

21. Li, Z.W.; Guo, C.; Nie, D.Y.; Lin, D.R.; Zhu, Y.; Chen, C.; Wu, X.H.; Xu, F.B.; Jin, C.J.; Zhang, X.Y.; et al. Deep learning for detecting retinal detachment and discerning macular status using ultra-widefield fundus images. *Commun. Biol.* **2020**, *3*, 15. [CrossRef]
22. Yan, Y.; Jin, K.; Gao, Z.; Huang, X.; Wang, F.; Wang, Y.; Ye, J. Attention-based deep learning system for automated diagnoses of age-related macular degeneration in optical coherence tomography images. *Med. Phys.* **2021**, *48*, 4926–4934. [CrossRef] [PubMed]
23. Gao, Z.; Jin, K.; Yan, Y.; Liu, X.; Shi, Y.; Ge, Y.; Pan, X.; Lu, Y.; Wu, J.; Wang, Y.; et al. End-to-end diabetic retinopathy grading based on fundus fluorescein angiography images using deep learning. *Graefes Arch. Clin. Exp. Ophthalmol.* **2022**, *260*, 1663–1673. [CrossRef] [PubMed]
24. Cao, J.; You, K.; Jin, K.; Lou, L.; Wang, Y.; Chen, M.; Pan, X.; Shao, J.; Su, Z.; Wu, J.; et al. Prediction of response to anti-vascular endothelial growth factor treatment in diabetic macular oedema using an optical coherence tomography-based machine learning method. *Acta Ophthalmol.* **2021**, *99*, e19–e27. [CrossRef] [PubMed]
25. Gu, H.; Guo, Y.W.; Gu, L.; Wei, A.J.; Xie, S.R.; Ye, Z.Q.; Xu, J.J.; Zhou, X.T.; Lu, Y.; Liu, X.Q.; et al. Deep learning for identifying corneal diseases from ocular surface slit-lamp photographs. *Sci. Rep.* **2020**, *10*, 17851. [CrossRef] [PubMed]
26. Tran, T.; Pham, T.; Carneiro, G.; Palmer, L.; Reid, I. A Bayesian Data Augmentation Approach for Learning Deep Models. In Proceedings of the Advances in Neural Information Processing Systems 30 (NIPS 2017), Long Beach, CA, USA, 4–9 December 2017.
27. Simonyan, K.; Zisserman, A.-P. Very Deep Convolutional Networks for Large-Scale Image Recognition. *arXiv* **2014**, arXiv:1409.1556.
28. Szegedy, C.; Liu, W.; Jia, Y.Q.; Sermanet, P.; Reed, S.; Anguelov, D.; Erhan, D.; Vanhoucke, V.; Rabinovich, A. Going Deeper with Convolutions. In Proceedings of the IEEE Conference on Computer Vision and Pattern Recognition, Boston, MA, USA, 7–12 June 2015; pp. 1–9.
29. Szegedy, C.; Ioffe, S.; Vanhoucke, V.; Alemi, A. Inception-v4, Inception-ResNet and the Impact of Residual Connections on Learning. *AAAI Conf. Artif. Intell.* **2016**, 31. [CrossRef]
30. Huang, G.; Liu, Z.; van der Maaten, L.; Weinberger, K.Q. Densely Connected Convolutional Networks. In Proceedings of the IEEE Conference on Computer Vision and Pattern Recognition, Honolulu, HI, USA, 21–26 July 2017; pp. 2261–2269.
31. Dosovitskiy, A.; Beyer, L.; Kolesnikov, A.; Weissenborn, D.; Zhai, X.; Unterthiner, T.; Dehghani, M.; Minderer, M.; Heigold, G.; Gelly, S.; et al. An Image is Worth 16x16 Words: Transformers for Image Recognition at Scale. *arXiv* **2020**, arXiv:2010.11929.
32. Tan, M.X.; Le, Q.V. EfficientNetV2: Smaller Models and Faster Training. In Proceedings of the International Conference on Machine Learning, Virtual, 18–24 July 2021; pp. 7102–7110.
33. Selvaraju, R.R.; Cogswell, M.; Das, A.; Vedantam, R.; Parikh, D.; Batra, D. Grad-CAM: Visual Explanations from Deep Networks via Gradient-based Localization. In Proceedings of the IEEE International Conference on Computer Vision, Venice, Italy, 22–29 October 2017; pp. 618–626.
34. Kuo, M.T.; Hsu, B.W.Y.; Yin, Y.K.; Fang, P.C.; Lai, H.Y.; Chen, A.; Yu, M.S.; Tseng, V.S. A deep learning approach in diagnosing fungal keratitis based on corneal photographs. *Sci. Rep.* **2020**, *10*, 14424. [CrossRef]
35. Ghosh, A.K.; Thammasudjarit, R.; Jongkhajornpong, P.; Attia, J.; Thakkinstian, A. Deep Learning for Discrimination Between Fungal Keratitis and Bacterial Keratitis: DeepKeratitis. *Cornea* **2022**, *41*, 616–622. [CrossRef]
36. Li, Z.W.; Jiang, J.W.; Chen, K.; Chen, Q.Q.; Zheng, Q.X.; Liu, X.T.; Weng, H.F.; Wu, S.J.; Chen, W. Preventing corneal blindness caused by keratitis using artificial intelligence. *Nat. Commun.* **2021**, *12*, 3738. [CrossRef]
37. Xu, Y.S.; Kong, M.; Xie, W.J.; Duan, R.P.; Fang, Z.Q.; Lin, Y.X.; Zhu, Q.; Tang, S.L.; Wu, F.; Yao, Y.F. Deep Sequential Feature Learning in Clinical Image Classification of Infectious Keratitis. *Engineering* **2021**, *7*, 1002–1010. [CrossRef]
38. Redd, T.K.; Prajna, N.V.; Srinivasan, M.; Lalitha, P.; Krishnan, T.; Rajaraman, R.; Venugopal, A.; Lujan, B.; Acharya, N.; Seitzman, G.D.; et al. Expert Performance in Visual Differentiation of Bacterial and Fungal Keratitis. *Ophthalmology* **2022**, *129*, 227–230. [CrossRef]
39. Yahya, G.; Ebada, A.; Khalaf, E.M.; Mansour, B.; Nouh, N.A.; Mosbah, R.A.; Saber, S.; Moustafa, M.; Negm, S.; El-Sokkary, M.M.A.; et al. Soil-Associated Bacillus Species: A Reservoir of Bioactive Compounds with Potential Therapeutic Activity against Human Pathogens. *Microorganisms* **2021**, *9*, 1131. [CrossRef]
40. El-Telbany, M.; Mohamed, A.A.; Yahya, G.; Abdelghafar, A.; Abdel-Halim, M.S.; Saber, S.; Alfaleh, M.A.; Mohamed, A.H.; Abdelrahman, F.; Fathey, H.A.; et al. Combination of Meropenem and Zinc Oxide Nanoparticles; Antimicrobial Synergism, Exaggerated Antibiofilm Activity, and Efficient Therapeutic Strategy against Bacterial Keratitis. *Antibiotics* **2022**, *11*, 1374. [CrossRef]

Journal of *Personalized Medicine*

MDPI

Article

Using the C-Read as a Portable Device to Evaluate Reading Ability in Young Chinese Adults: An Observational Study

Tian Cheng [1,†], Taikang Yao [1,†], Boxuan Xu [1], Wanwei Dai [2,3], Xuejiao Qin [4], Juan Ye [5], Lingge Suo [2,3,*] and Chun Zhang [2,3]

1 Peking University Health Science Center, Peking University, Beijing 100191, China
2 Department of Ophthalmology, Peking University Third Hospital, Beijing 100191, China
3 Beijing Key Laboratory of Restoration of Damaged Ocular Nerve, Peking University Third Hospital, Beijing 100191, China
4 Department of Ophthalmology, The Second Hospital of Shandong University, Jinan 250033, China
5 Department of Ophthalmology, The Second Affiliated Hospital Zhejiang University, Hangzhou 310058, China
* Correspondence: suolingge_1019@126.com; Tel.: +86-15529527020
† These authors contributed equally to this work.

Abstract: We evaluated the reading characteristics of normal-sighted young adults using C-Read to provide baseline healthy population values. We also investigated the relationship between the National Eye Institute's Visual Functioning Questionnaire (VFQ-25) score and reading ability, myopia, and hours of screen use, focusing on the extent to which these factors affect participants' visual function and, ultimately, their vision-related quality of life (QoL). Overall, 207 young, healthy participants (414 eyes) aged 18–35 years were tested for reading speed using C-Read connected to a smartphone-based application between December 2022 and January 2023. Each participant received a VFQ-25 questionnaire to evaluate vision-related QoL. Data on daily e-screen usage hours were collected. Among the participants, 91 (44.0%) were women; their mean (SD) age was 22.45 (4.01) years. The mean (SD) reading acuity (RA) was 0.242 (0.124), 0.249 (0.120), and 0.193 (0.104) logarithmic minimum angle of resolution (logMAR) for the right, left, and both eyes, respectively. The mean (SD) maximum reading speed (MRS) was 171.65 (46.27), 168.59 (45.68), and 185.16 (44.93) words per minute (wpm) with the right, left, and both eyes, respectively. The mean (SD) critical print size (CPS) was 0.412 (0.647), 0.371 (0.229), and 0.419 (1.05) logMAR per the right, left, and both eyes, respectively. The RA and CPS were significantly different between sexes (p = 0.002 and p = 0.001). MRS was significantly different between the education level (p = 0.005) and myopia level groups (p = 0.010); however, it was not clear whether this difference was confounded by age. The myopic power in diopters significantly affected RA (coefficient, −0.012; 95% CI, −0.018 to −0.006; p = 0.001), screen time significantly affected MRS (coefficient, 0.019, 95% CI, 0.57 to 6.33, p = 0.019). RA (coefficient, −21.41; 95% CI, −33.74 to −9.08; p = 0.001) and duration of screen use (coefficient, −0.86; 95% CI, −1.29 to −0.43; p < 0.001) independently had a significantly negative correlation with VFQ-25 scores. Our findings provide a baseline value for C-Read in normal-sighted young adults. Refractive status significantly affected RA, while screen time significantly affected MRS. Interventions aimed at enhancing RA may have the potential to maximize vision-related QoL and enable older adults with impaired vision to achieve greater outcomes. Future, larger-scale, C-Read experiments will help provide newer, more optimal methods for the early diagnosis of visual impairment.

Keywords: C-Read; reading speed; smartphone-based application; healthy subjects

Citation: Cheng, T.; Yao, T.; Xu, B.; Dai, W.; Qin, X.; Ye, J.; Suo, L.; Zhang, C. Using the C-Read as a Portable Device to Evaluate Reading Ability in Young Chinese Adults: An Observational Study. *J. Pers. Med.* **2023**, *13*, 463. https://doi.org/10.3390/jpm13030463

Academic Editor: Jiawei Zhou

Received: 10 January 2023
Revised: 22 February 2023
Accepted: 27 February 2023
Published: 1 March 2023

1. Introduction

Reading is a core function of vision. Currently, the epidemic increase in the prevalence of myopia among school-aged children and the increase in the number of older adults with age-related conditions (e.g., presbyopia, glaucoma, age-related macular degeneration) contribute to challenging public health conditions worldwide [1]. It is projected that by

2050 half of the world's population will be myopic [2]. There is conclusive evidence that visual impairment can lead to reading difficulty and directly affect quality of life (QoL) [3]. However, the relationship between myopia and reading is less adequately studied, although myopia is a risk factor for visual impairment. Kandel et al. [4] pointed out that myopia can cause difficulties in reading, driving, sports, and entertainment activities, which in turn reduce quality of life.

According to a large study of children and adults of all ages, 62% of patients seeking low-vision consultation were primarily interested in improving their reading ability [5]. Reading ability is often used as an outcome indicator in clinical trials to assess the effectiveness of treatments, surgical procedures, and rehabilitation techniques [6–8]. In addition, reading ability is easy and inexpensive to assess and can be administered outside the hospital. It is, therefore, an appropriate choice for early self-testing.

Numerous continuous-text reading-ability tests have been developed and applied in vision health care, most notably the Minnesota Low-Vision Reading Test (MNREAD) [9,10] and Radner Reading charts [11,12]. Both tests quantify reading ability by measuring three core reading ability indicators [13]: reading acuity (RA): the smallest print that can just be read; maximum reading speed (MRS): the reading speed when performance is not limited by print size; and critical print size (CPS): the smallest print that supports the maximum reading speed. However, the MNREAD and Radner Reading charts are available only in English, limiting the application of these scales in non-English-speaking countries.

Han et al. [14] developed and validated the Chinese reading-ability test chart, C-Read, and its supporting electronic portable device to assess Chinese reading ability. There are three scales in C-Read, each consisting of 16 12-character simplified Chinese sentences acquired from first- to third-grade textbooks, and they have been tested for homogeneity [14]. The C-Read derives some time-tested design principles from the aforementioned tests, including the standardized continuous text that closely resembles daily reading materials, high-frequency vocabulary at the primary reading level, the most streamlined typefaces, logarithmic progression of print sizes, and consistency in the spatial arrangement of sentences [10,15]. In addition, given the many differences between logographic Chinese and linear alphabetic Latin languages, such as sentence composition, the number of syllables, and the use of Chinese characters with simple and complex strokes, C-Read adapted the above design principles based on an in-depth understanding of these features of Chinese text reading [14]. The reliability of the C-Read has also been tested using passages from the International Reading Speed Text (IReST) [16]; the results showed that C-Read scores could accurately predict passage reading ability over a wide range of refractions [17]. Hence, this indicated that C-Read is a reliable and valid clinical tool for quantitatively assessing the reading ability of readers of simplified Chinese characters.

Another major advantage of C-Read is that it allows continuous-text reading ability tests on an electronic screen. This advantage facilitates data processing and meets the increasing reality of digital reading for citizens in the 21st century [18]. Digital versions of reading tests are also advantageous because text size, contrast polarity, color, and font size can be easily adjusted. However, the performance of any digital reading test largely depends on screen size, display technology, and resolution [19]. MNREAD and Radner reading tests have been shown to have minimal differences between the evaluation parameters of the digital and traditional versions [2,20–22]. Therefore, it is dependable to use electronic devices for reading-ability tests.

Little is known about the reading characteristics of young adults with normal vision whose native language is Chinese, due to the lack of a reliable Chinese reading chart to assess Chinese reading ability. Han et al. [14] measured the reading characteristics of 118 Chinese college students between the ages of 18–24 who had normal or corrected vision and obtained normal mean (SD) reference values for RA, CPS, and MRS of 0.16 (0.05) logMAR, 0.24 (0.06) logMAR, and 273.44 (34.37) Chinese wpm, respectively. In addition, previous studies have observed a clear correlation between reading speed and vision-related QoL in people with eye disease, and the results of a study by an Italian academic [23] point to both reading speed and visual acuity as important determinants of quality of life. However, it remains to be seen whether this correlation holds in the healthy population. The objectives of this study were (1) to evaluate the reading characteristics of normally sighted young adults over a wider age range (18–35 years) using a C-Read test to provide baseline values in young Chinese adults, and (2) to investigate the relationship between the VFQ-25 scale and reading ability, myopia, and screen-use hours in young Chinese adults, looking at how these factors affect visual function and, ultimately, vision-related QoL.

2. Materials and Methods

2.1. Study Design

This single-center observational study was approved by the Institutional Review Board of Peking University Third Hospital (IRB00006761-M2022800) and followed the tenets of the Declaration of Helsinki. Informed consent was obtained from all participants after the experimental procedures were fully described. The trial was registered with the Chinese Clinical Trial Registry (NCT5673954) and followed the Consolidated Standards of Reporting Trials (CONSORT) reporting guidelines.

2.2. Participants

Figure 1 shows the flow diagram of the participants according to the CONSORT statement [24]. We set $\sigma = 7\delta$ and $\alpha = 0.05$, ran a two-sided test, and worked out that the sample needed 189 people. Considering a 5% missing rate, a total of at least 200 people needed to be recruited at first. In total, 219 healthy participants were recruited for this study at Peking University between December 2022 and January 2023. To reduce selection bias due to non-random willingness to participate in the survey, participants were recruited by simple random sampling from different academic departments at Peking University (including Humanities, Science, Social Sciences, and Medicine). Healthy participants were included according to the following criteria: (1) age between 18 and 35 years; (2) best-corrected visual acuity (BCVA) $\geq$1.0 decimal by using standard logarithmic visual acuity chart; (3) good physiological functioning of the body's systems without health problems requiring medical intervention; (4) no strabismus, amblyopia, or any other ocular or systemic diseases that may affect reading ability; (5) good cooperation in the questionnaire survey and reading tests. Professional ophthalmologists examined the subjects for distance and near vision via slit lamp observation and indirect ophthalmoscopy. All subjects' eye health status was confirmed by professional ophthalmologists.

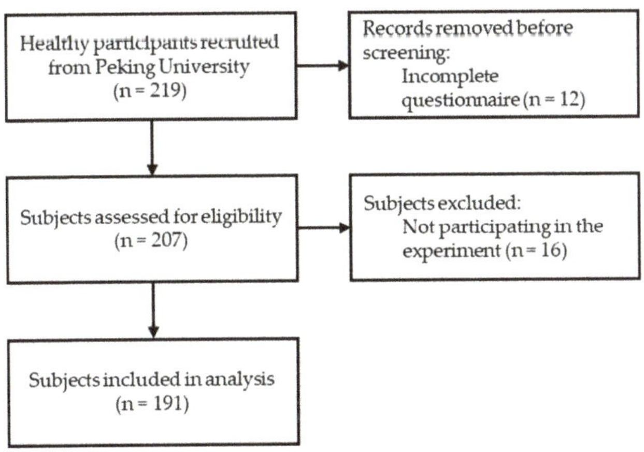

Figure 1. Flow Diagram of Participants According to CONSORT Statement.

2.3. Screen Time and Visual QoL

A questionnaire was designed to collect the participants' sex, age, refractive status, and time spent on screens, including personal computers, phones, and pads (see Supplementary Materials). Furthermore, the VFQ-25 [25] was chosen to collect and assess visual QoL. The VFQ-25 is a reliable questionnaire used to evaluate vision-related QoL globally [26–30]. It has 12 subscales that cover general health, general vision, eye pain, near activities, distance activities, social functioning, mental health, role difficulties, dependency, driving, color vision, and peripheral vision. In this study, the Chinese version of the VFQ-25 developed by Chan et al., was used [30].

2.4. C-Read Device and Smartphone-Based App

The procedure is illustrated in Figure 2. The C-Read test was performed in a well-lit room with the device placed on a special stand that was vertically fixed at eye level. The mean screen luminance of the C-Read device is 150–250 cd/m^2. The participants sat 40 cm from the screen, with their heads on the headrest, verbally reading sentences from the screen's top row (largest print size). They were instructed to read these sentences as fast as possible without making any errors and encouraged to read as many characters as possible when encountering sentences with smaller print sizes. In addition, a triangular guide symbol appeared on the screen at the beginning of each sentence indicating their location. The test was stopped when the participants reported that they could no longer read any character.

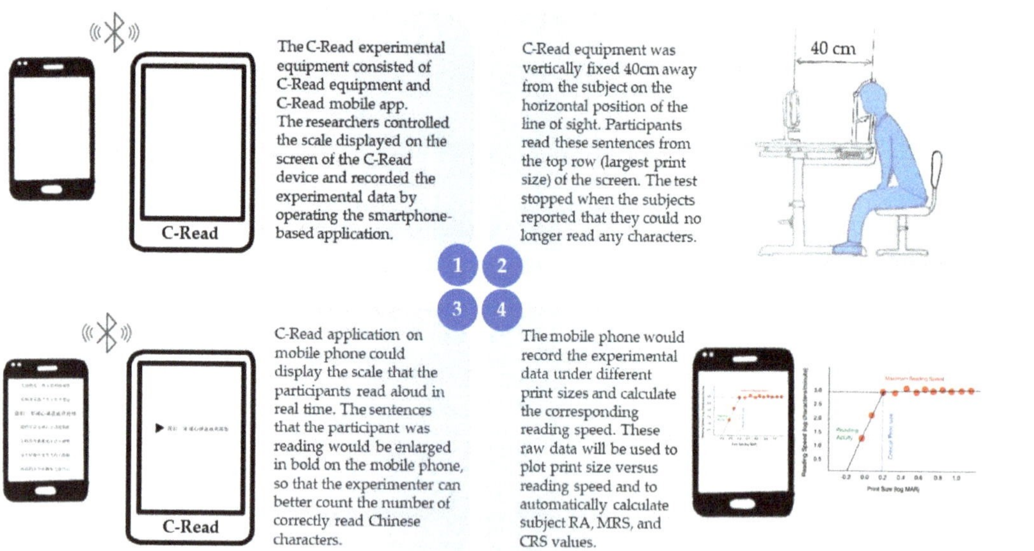

Figure 2. Flow Diagram of Trial Design. Abbreviations: RA, reading acuity; MRS, maximum reading speed; CPS, critical print size.

The C-Read application on the smartphone recorded the time each participant spent reading the sentences aloud and the number of correct Chinese characters read. The C-Read application on the phone was connected to the C-Read device using Bluetooth. Three scales, A, B, and C, were used to assess participants' binocular, right-eye, and left-eye reading ability. We used scale A to test both eyes; scale B to test the left eye; scale C to test the right eye. When changing eyes, the examiner could switch to a different scale for the next test using the C-Read application on the smartphone (see Figures S1 and S2).

The measuring principle of C-Read was as follows: the reading speed vs. print size curves obtained in the C-Read test for normal and low-vision subjects have the same typical shape [9]. Over a wide range of print sizes, the reading speed remains constant, forming a platform representative of MRS. When the print size reaches a certain value and the reading speed decreases rapidly, the print size is called CPS. The minimum print size that can be read is defined as the RA. C-Read used a hybrid algorithm to obtain the reading characteristics, that is, using a bilinear fitting algorithm to determine the critical character size and maximum reading speed and using the MNREAD method to calculate RA [14].

The smartphone uploaded all the experimental data (the number of Chinese characters correctly read and the time spent reading them) under different print sizes, recorded in the C-Read application program, to the cloud storage and calculated the corresponding reading speeds under different print sizes. These raw data were used to plot the print size versus reading speed graph, and the program automatically calculated the RA, MRS, and CRS values. The participants' reading abilities could be assessed by analyzing these reading characteristics.

2.5. Data Collection and Statistical Analysis

All questionnaires were collected after obtaining informed consent from the subjects. The researcher briefed the participants on the purpose and methods of the experiment. Most of the information was collected as completed online questionnaires, and some of it was collected using paper questionnaires. Data from all questionnaires carefully completed by the participants were included in the analysis.

Data analysis was performed using the STATA Statistics Software (Version 17.0; Stata Corp., College Station, Texas, USA). Figures were drawn using GraphPad Prism (version 7.0; GraphPad Software, Inc., San Diego, CA, USA). The distribution of the variables was judged using Kolmogorov–Smirnov test. Mann–Whitney test and Kruskal–Wallis test were used to analyze differences in reading ability between gender, education, and myopia levels. Factors affecting reading ability and the relationship between reading ability and QoL were analyzed using multiple linear regression models and stepwise adjustment. Statistical significance was set at $p < 0.05$.

3. Results

3.1. Demographics

In total, 219 healthy participants were surveyed. Finally, 207 participants returned the completed questionnaire, resulting in a response rate of 94.5% (207/219). The age range of the participants who met the eligibility criteria was 18–35 (median, 21 years; interquartile range, 19–24 years).

Among the 207 participants, 91 (44.0%) were female, and the mean (SD) age was 22.45 (4.01). Participant characteristics are listed in Table 1. Myopia between −0.00 and −0.50 diopters is classified as emmetropia. Low, moderate, and high myopia describe myopia between −0.50 and −3.00, −3.00 and −6.00, −6.00 or more diopters, respectively [31]. All participants were native Chinese speakers. None of the studies had gender restrictions on sampling; therefore, the unequal number of males and females reflects the nature of the volunteers.

Table 1. Baseline characteristics of participants in this study.

Characteristic	No. (%)
	Healthy Group (n = 207)
Age, mean (SD), y	22.46 (4.01)
Gender	
Male	116 (56.04)
Female	91 (43.96)

Table 1. *Cont.*

Characteristic	No. (%)
	Healthy Group (n = 207)
Education	
Undergraduate	146 (71.22)
Postgraduate	26 (12.68)
Doctor and Postdoc	33 (16.10)
Myopia, eyes	
No	40 (9.66)
Low	144 (34.78)
Moderate	187 (45.17)
High	43 (10.39)
Screen time, mean (SD), h	
Phone	4.55 (1.37)
Personal computer	4.32 (1.65)
Pad	2.55 (1.71)
Total	5.06 (1.50)
VFQ-25, mean (SD)	86.26 (9.11)

Abbreviations: VFQ, visual functioning questionnaire.

3.2. Characteristics of Reading Speed

Table 2 shows the participants' reading characteristics. The mean (SD) RA for the young, healthy population was 0.242 (0.124), 0.249 (0.120), and 0.193 (0.104) logMAR in the right, left, and both eyes, respectively. The mean (SD) MRS for the young, healthy population was 171.65 (46.27), 168.59 (45.68), and 185.16 (44.93) wpm in the right, left, and both eyes, respectively. The mean (SD) CPS for the young, healthy population was 0.412 (0.647), 0.371 (0.229), and 0.419 (1.05) logMAR in the right, left, and both eyes, respectively. Figure 3 shows the reading characteristics for both, left, and right eyes for different sexes, education levels, and myopia levels. We found that RA and CPS significantly differed between the sex groups (Figure 3a,c; $p = 0.005$, $p = 0.025$). CPS showed a significant difference among the myopia groups (Table 3; $p < 0.001$) in a single eye and tended to increase with myopia progression (Figure 3i). In addition, MRS was statistically different between the education groups (Table 3; $p = 0.002$), but it was unclear whether this difference was confounded by age. We also analyzed the data from the left and right eyes mixed together as a single eye and obtained exactly the same results (see Figure S3).

Table 2. Reading characteristics of participants in this study.

Characteristic	Mean (SD)
	Healthy Group (n = 191)
RA, logMAR	
both eyes	0.193 (0.104)
right eye	0.242 (0.124)
left eye	0.249 (0.120)
MRS, wpm	
both eyes	185.16 (44.93)
right eye	171.65 (46.27)
left eye	168.59 (45.68)
CPS, logMAR	
both eyes	0.419 (1.05)
right eye	0.412 (0.647)
left eye	0.371 (0.229)

Abbreviations: RA, reading acuity; MAR, minimum angle of resolution; MRS, maximum reading speed; wpm, words per minute; CPS, critical print size.

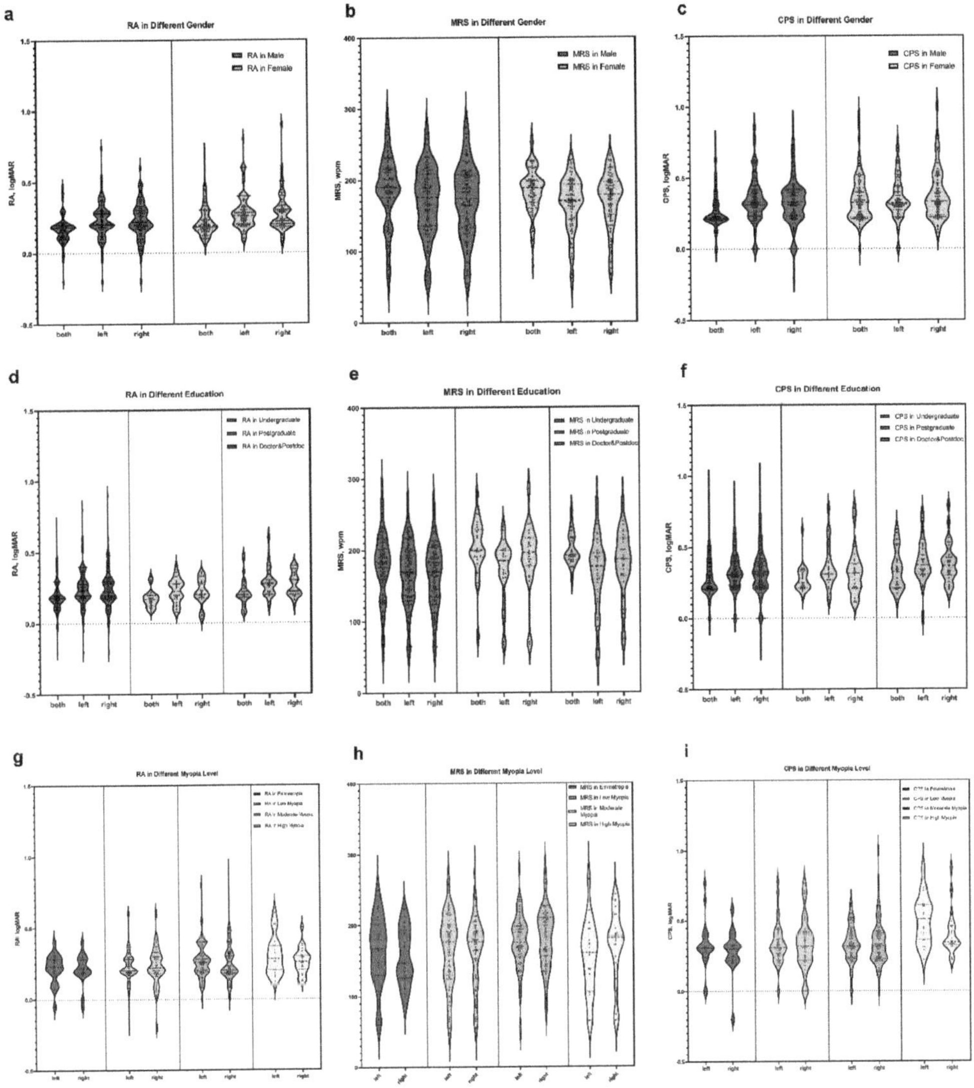

Figure 3. Reading characteristics for both, left, and right eyes for different sexes, education levels, and myopia levels. (**a**) The RA for different sexes was statistically significant ($n = 191$, $p = 0.005$), as determined by the two-tailed Mann–Whitney test. (**b**) The MRS for different sexes was not statistically different ($n = 191$, $p = 0.685$), as determined by the two-tailed Mann–Whitney test. (**c**) The CPS for different sexes was statistically significant ($n = 191$, $p = 0.025$), as determined by the two-tailed Mann–Whitney test. (**d**) The RA of the three education levels was not significantly different ($n = 189$, $p = 0.217$), as determined by the Kruskal–Wallis test. (**e**) The MRS for the three education levels was statistically significant ($n = 189$, $p = 0.002$), as determined by the Kruskal–Wallis test. (**f**) The CPS for different education levels was not statistically different ($n = 189$, $p = 0.093$), as determined by the Kruskal–Wallis test. (**g**) The RA for the different myopia levels was not statistically significant ($n = 382$ eyes, $p = 0.072$), as determined by the Kruskal–Wallis test. (**h**) The MRS for different myopia levels was statistically significant ($n = 382$ eyes, $p = 0.049$), as determined by the Kruskal–Wallis test. (**i**) The CPS for different myopia levels was statistically significant ($n = 382$ eyes, $p < 0.001$), as determined by the Kruskal–Wallis test. Abbreviations: RA, reading acuity; MRS, maximum reading speed; CPS, critical print size.

Table 3. Left- and right-eye reading characteristics for different genders, education levels, and myopia levels.

		RA	MRS	CPS
Gender	Male (n = 105)	0.17 (0.10)	184.95 (52.74)	0.27 (0.13)
	Female (n = 86)	0.22 (0.11)	185.42 (33.29)	0.34 (0.15)
	p value	0.005	0.685	0.025
Education	Undergraduate (n = 133)	0.19 (0.11)	178.57 (48.40)	0.30 (0.15)
	Postgraduate (n = 26)	0.17 (0.06)	203.76 (39.07)	0.27 (0.09)
	Doctor and Postdoc (n = 30)	0.21 (0.10)	199.64 (21.80)	0.33 (0.14)
	p value	0.217	0.002	0.093
Myopia	No (n = 37)	0.16 (0.08)	162.4 (42.9)	0.29 (0.10)
	Low (n = 136)	0.19 (0.11)	163.2 (46.1)	0.34 (0.15)
	Moderate (n = 166)	0.19 (0.11)	178.6 (43.4)	0.34 (0.14)
	High (n = 43)	0.22 (0.08)	162.9 (44.7)	0.44 (0.18)
	p value	0.772	0.049	< 0.001

Abbreviations: RA, reading acuity; MRS, maximum reading speed; CPS, critical print size.

3.3. *Effect of Age, Myopia, and Screen Time on Reading Ability*

Table 4 shows the multivariate linear regression model for the correlation between monocular reading characteristics, age, screen time, and monocular myopic refraction in diopters. After adjustment using stepwise regression, we found that the myopic power had a significant effect on RA (Figure 4a; coefficient, −0.012; 95% CI, −0.018 to −0.006; p = 0.001), screen time had a significant effect on MRS (Figure 4b; coefficient, 0.019; 95% CI, 0.57 to 6.33; p = 0.019), and both myopic refraction (diopters) and screen time had a significant effect on CPS (Figure 4c; diopters: coefficient, 0.015; 95% CI, 0.004 to 0.026; p < 0.001; screen time: coefficient, −0.014; 95% CI, −0.021 to −0.006; p = 0.010). Parameter estimates for the MLR models of RA, MRS, and CPS for right, left, and both eyes are presented in Table S1. However, since the participants recruited in this research were all young, healthy people, the insignificance of age does not mean that age does not affect these reading characteristics.

Table 4. Parameter estimates for multivariate linear regression model of RA, MRS, and CPS in a single eye.

Measure		Multivariate Linear Regression		Stepwise Regression (p value = 0.05)	
		β (95% CI)	p Value	β (95% CI)	p Value
RA	Intercept	0.213 (0.128 to 0.297)	<0.001	0.22 (0.19 to 0.24)	<0.001
	Age, y	−0.00074 (−0.00387 to 0.00239)	0.642		
	Screen time, h	0.0044 (−0.0045 to 0.0133)	0.331		
	Myopia, D	−0.012 (−0.018 to −0.006)	<0.001	−0.012 (−0.018 to −0.006)	<0.001
MRS	Intercept	179.77 (152.39 to 207.15)	<0.001	166.0 (150.9 to 181.1)	<0.001
	Age, y	−0.55 (−1.56 to 0.47)	0.289		
	Screen time, h	3.45 (0.57 to 6.33)	0.019	3.19 (0.34 to 6.04)	0.028
	Myopia, D	0.68 (−1.33 to 2.69)	0.507		
CPS	Intercept	0.19 (0.09 to 0.30)	<0.001	0.23 (0.16 to 0.29)	<0.001
	Age, y	−0.0014 (−0.024 to 0.005)	0.467		
	Screen time, h	0.015 (0.004 to 0.026)	0.010	0.015 (0.004 to 0.026)	0.007
	Myopia, D	−0.013 (−0.021 to −0.006)	<0.001	−0.013 (−0.021 to −0.006)	<0.001

Abbreviations: D, diopter; RA, reading acuity; MRS, maximum reading speed; CPS, critical print size.

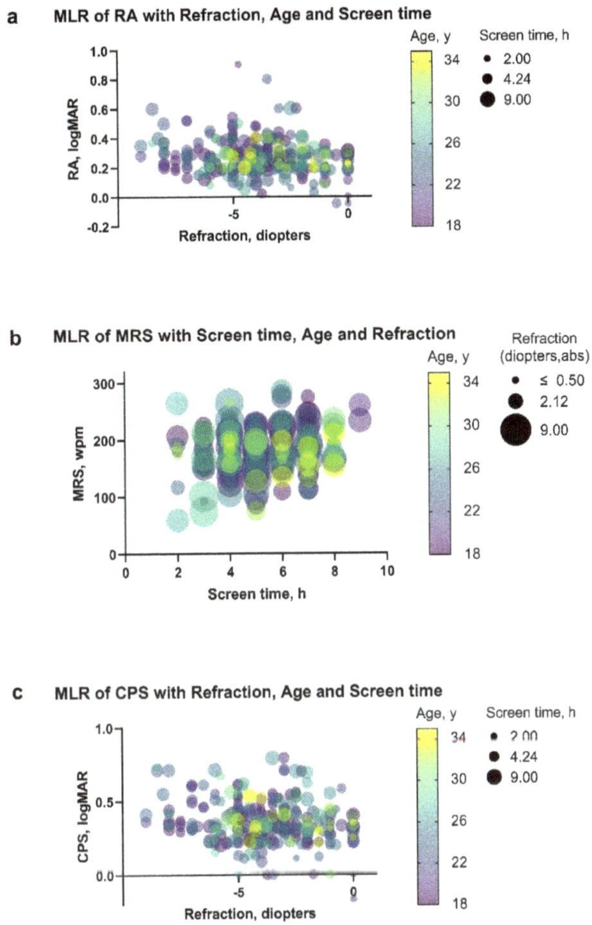

Figure 4. Parameter estimates for multivariate linear regression model for the outcomes RA, MRS, and CPS. (**a**) RA as a function of myopic power, age, and screen time. Points show both eyes' RA for each participant tested. The age of participants is color-coded, and the screen time is size-coded. (**b**) MRS as a function of screen time, age, and refraction (diopters). Points show both eyes' MRS for each participant tested. The ages of participants are color-coded, and the myopic power of participants is size coded. (**c**) CPS as a function of refraction (diopters), age, and screen time. Points show both eyes' CPS for each participant tested. The age of participants is color-coded, and the screen time is size-coded. Model estimates and their 95% CI are given in Table 4. Abbreviations: abs, absolute value; MLR, multiple linear regression; RA, reading acuity; MRS, maximum reading speed; CPS, critical print size.

3.4. Effect of Reading Ability on VFQ-25 Score Results

Reading is an important part of visual life, and a decline in the reading function directly impacts a patient's QoL. While clinicians are primarily concerned with changes in pathological factors, patients are interested in how these factors affect their functional status and vision-related QoL. The VFQ-25 is used to measure the vision-specific quality of life, such as stereoacuity, light adaptation, and dark adaptation, and to evaluate the overall quality of survival states, including self-care, activity, and social and psychological parameters.

Figure 5 shows the regressions of VFQ-25 scores using data from the right, left, and both eyes. The independent variables included age; visual acuity; the amount of time spent on computers, phones, and pads; and three criteria of reading ability. Furthermore, using a stepwise adjustment process, two significant independent variables were selected: RA (Table 5; coefficient, −21.41; 95% CI, −33.74 to −9.08; $p = 0.001$) and the duration of screen use (Table 5; coefficient, −0.86; 95% CI, −1.29 to −0.43; $p < 0.001$). Both had negative correlation coefficients with VFQ-25 scores, which could be explained by the fact that longer screen time would lead to a greater impact on vision-related functions. In addition, a larger RA value would indicate a greater decline in visual acuity, which could also contribute to a lower VFQ-25 score.

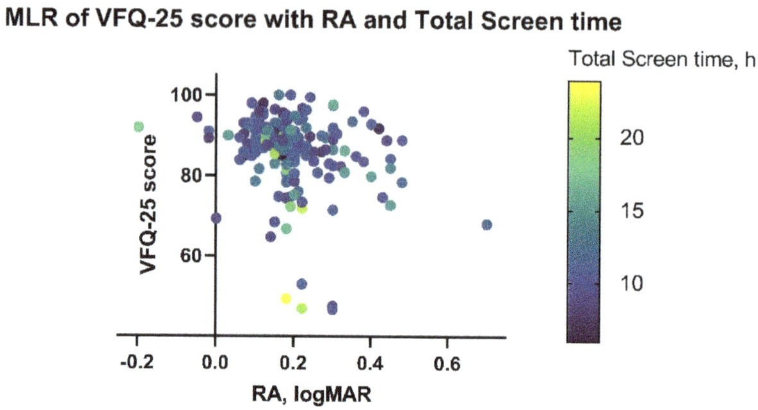

Figure 5. Parameter estimates for multivariate linear regression model for VFQ-25 score outcomes. The VFQ-25 score is significantly correlated with RA and the amount of screen time. Points show the VFQ-25 score for each participant assessed. The amount of screen time of participants is color-coded. Abbreviations: VFQ, visual functioning questionnaire.

Table 5. Parameter estimates for multivariate linear regression and stepwise regression model for the outcomes VFQ-25 score.

Measure		Multivariate Linear Regression		Stepwise Regression (p Value = 0.05)	
		β (95% CI)	p Value	β (95% CI)	p Value
Right eye	Intercept	109.76 (99.15 to 120.38)	<0.001	100.82 (94.78 to 106.86)	<0.001
	Age, y	−0.17 (−0.50 to 0.15)	0.298		
	Total screen time, h	−0.86 (−1.30 to −0.42)	<0.001	−0.86 (−1.29 to −0.42)	<0.001
	Refraction, D	0.42 (−0.17 to 1.01)	0.164		
	RA, logMAR	−16.60 (−32.19 to −1.00)	0.037	−18.65 (−30.88 to −6.43)	0.003
	MRS, wpm	−0.017 (−0.046 to 0.012)	0.240		
	CPS, logMAR	−2.75 (−14.36 to 8.86)	0.640		
Left eye	Intercept	105.58 (95.57 to 115.60)	<0.001	100.68 (95.15 to 106.21)	<0.001
	Age, y	−0.08 (−0.37 to 0.21)	0.598		
	Total screen time, h	−0.64 (−1.05 to −0.23)	0.002	−0.63 (−1.04 to −0.23)	0.002
	Refraction, D	0.11 (−0.43 to 0.65)	0.683		
	RA, logMAR	−21.31 (−35.69 to −6.92)	0.004	−26.83 (−37.84 to −15.83)	<0.001
	MRS, wpm	−0.01 (−0.04 to 0.02)	0.429		
	CPS, logMAR	−6.28 (−17.37 to 4.82)	0.266		
Both eyes *	Intercept	107.25 (96.62 to 117.89)	<0.001	100.24 (94.59 to 105.89)	<0.001
	Age, y	−0.12 (−0.44 to 0.20)	0.451		
	Total screen time, h	−0.88 (−1.32 to −0.44)	<0.001	−0.86 (−1.29 to −0.43)	<0.001
	RA, logMAR	−15.61 (−30.70 to −0.52)	0.043	−21.41 (−33.74 to −9.08)	0.001
	MRS, wpm	−0.015 (−0.045 to 0.015)	0.330		
	CPS, logMAR	−7.59 (−18.30 to 3.12)	0.164		

Abbreviations: D, diopter; RA, reading acuity; MAR, minimum angle of resolution; MRS, maximum reading speed; wpm, words per minute; CPS, critical print size; VFQ, visual functioning questionnaire. *: Refraction was not included in the regression model for both eyes since refraction was not significant for VFQ-25 scores in both the left and right eyes.

4. Discussion

Reading performance predicts visual ability and vision-related QoL [32]. Although there is no consensus on the best way to assess reading performance, most tests have identified a common set of characteristics [32]: (i) MRS and RA are key outcome variables, while tests of comprehension or reading stamina are reserved for specific research questions; (ii) reading speed is measured for meaningful text, although this may allow cognitive factors to have a greater impact; and (iii) to ensure that the text is read accurately, reading aloud rather than silently is preferred. Reading aloud also facilitates scoring [33].

In 1854, Jaeger invented the Near Vision Scale, marking the first clinical reading test [34]. In the century and a half that followed, dozens of reading-ability tests appeared, but there were few Chinese versions of these tests. In addition to the C-Read from MNREAD, the only other tests are the IResT, which was translated into 19 languages, including Chinese by Klosinski et al. [35] in 2012, and the Chinese reading-speed test for children by Cheung et al. [36] in 2015. Few studies of these Chinese-language tests were based on smartphone applications, which measure close-reading ability.

With technology advancement, more tests with multiple functions to assess close-reading ability were used, and the widely accepted ones included MNREAD and IReST. In general, IReST is more advantageous for measuring reading speed for fixed print sizes [35], and the MNREAD Acuity Test is widely used for measuring reading speed for texts of different sizes [32]. The Chinese version of the reading speed scale C-Read was developed on the basis of MNREAD. It used sentences of a standardized reading level and length, acquired the reliability and stability of the MNREAD test, and had good test repeatability, making it a reliable measure of Chinese reading ability [14]. Moreover, through improvements in the medium, C-Read could support testing on higher-resolution e-readers via a smartphone-based application, which is certainly more relevant nowadays as e-reading time is significantly longer.

Notably, a "floor effect" is frequently observed in the C-Read test. Here, participants can only correctly read one or two characters per sentence of the two or three smallest characters before they stop trying, resulting in a floor effect at the small-character-size end of the reading speed graph [37]. This effect may be unique to simplified Chinese reading because of the presence of simple and readable characters in these sentences. To correct the effect caused by the floor effect, the C-Read program automatically removes all characters in the floor effect except for the largest character in size, producing a monotonically rising linear part of the reading speed function used to calculate the C-Read parameter [14].

Reading performance is one of the most important outcome indicators of the effectiveness of therapeutic interventions and vision rehabilitation. Despite the many differences between highly standardized clinical reading tests and daily reading, clinical test scores are good predictors of reading ability [38]. We aimed to assess the performance of university students with normal vision in the C-Read test, providing baseline values for that test in a healthy population. Our reference values for reading characteristics in the healthy young population were lower than those of Han et al. [14]. This may be due to the inclusion of a wider age range in our participants, particularly those over 30 years old. This finding also reinforces the strong association between reading ability and age.

Reading characteristics provide interesting insights into the functional performance of patients before and after therapy. However, we expected them to be used more frequently as an early screening test for vision loss disorders. Most visual function questionnaires ask patients to self-report assessments of their reading difficulties. Although self-reported ability is usually consistent with measured reading performance, there can be discrepancies, especially when patients self-perceive no reading difficulties but test results indicate RA or MRS impairment. This inconsistency between self-perception and examination results may indicate preclinical visual impairment and requires further examination [39].

Another project explored the relationship between the time spent on electronic screens and reading characteristics. We chose college students because the prevalence of myopia among college students is high and they tend to be younger [40–42]. Students are also extensive users of electronic devices, and their exposure to screen terminals is increasing and diversifying. Notably, online learning during home isolation after the COVID-19 outbreak has significantly prolonged the electronic screen exposure of college students [17,43]. These students faced a huge visual burden, leading to eye fatigue, blurred vision, eye dryness, or myopia [44–46]. However, the relationship between screen-viewing behavior and myopia is unclear or even contradictory [42,47–49]. A plausible reason is that the existing research on screen-viewing behavior is not sufficiently accurate and comprehensive, and the evaluation methods have difficulty considering the intensity and duration of screen use.

Our study initially revealed that the myopic power is a key factor affecting RA, presumably because both are physical quantities indicating visual acuity. The negative correlation coefficient between screen time and MRS can be well explained by the fact that long-duration eye use causes eye strain, reducing reading speed. CPS is associated with both myopic power and screen time, which reflected the joint effect of visual acuity and eye strain on the turning point in close reading. In addition, Calabrèse et al. [50] pointed out that age was also related to reading characteristics; however, due to the age limit of this study, we did not find a significant correlation between age and reading characteristics.

RA and CPS showed significant differences between sex groups. The significant differences in RA and CPS between sex groups may reflect differences in eye-tracking habits between women and men. Our study found that women spent an average of 0.73 h (11.78 for women and 11.05 h for men, $p = 0.040$) more time using screens daily than men and that longer screen use may account for the lower average RA and CPS in women than in men (see Figure S4). The differences in MRS scores between the education and myopia arrays were significant. Although it was unclear whether this difference was affected by age, it might reflect, to some extent, the influence of education and learning experience on reading ability. Both RA and CPS increased with myopia level; however, the difference among the various myopia level groups was insignificant, which might be related to the insufficient sample size.

Two variables, RA and the amount of screen time, had negative correlation coefficients with VFQ-25 scores. We collected both participants' subjective perceived screen time and objective daily personal computer, phone, and pad usage time, finding that the latter negatively affected the visual QoL, whereas the former had no such effect. Chan et al. [51] reported that the visual acuity of the better eye is highly correlated with the quality of life. As mentioned above, longer screen exposure predisposes patients to myopia with decreased RA, whereas deterioration in visual function may result in a lower VFQ-25 score. We also observed that the VFQ-25 score gradually decreased with an increase in myopia level, which is consistent with previous studies (see Table S3, Figure S5c) [52]. There was no significant difference in VFQ-25 scores between the sexes.

Zhu et al. [52] found that educational attainment was also an important demographic factor affecting the VFQ-25 score because patients with higher educational attainment might know more about eye conditions and seek suitable treatment before irreversible damage occurs. It has been reported that knowledge of eye diseases is an important positive predictor of QoL [53]. However, in this study, no significant difference was observed between educational level and VFQ-25 score, which might be because the subjects participating in the study were all well-educated college students.

The limitation of this study is the lack of age-related controls. The subjects in this study were all in the 18–35 age group and there were no data for children or middle-aged or elderly healthy subjects, which may explain why we did not observe a negative correlation between VFQ-25 score and age. Further experiments covering subjects with wider age ranges to explore the effect of age on reading characteristics and visual QoL are necessary. However, our study initially investigated the negative correlation between screen time and RA and VFQ-25 scores, which led us to question whether long-term electronic screen use has an impact on eye health consequences and whether there is a time point beyond which visual health deteriorates rapidly with screen use.

5. Conclusions

Our findings provide baseline values for C-Read in healthy individuals. Myopic power was a significant factor affecting RA, while screen-use time significantly affected MRS. CPS was associated with both myopic power and screen time. In addition, RA and CPS significantly differed between sex groups, increasing with the progression of myopia. Finally, MRS scores were significantly different between different education and myopia level groups.

A person's RA can significantly affect their vision-related QoL, suggesting that interventions aimed at enhancing RA might have the potential to maximize visual quality. This would enable some older adults with impaired vision to achieve better outcomes from low-vision rehabilitation. Total screen time negatively affected vision-related QoL, although participants perceived that screen-use time had no such effect. More research is needed to investigate the relationship between RA, screen time, and vision-related QoL.

Reading performance is an important indicator of reactive visual functioning. A significant difference between a patient's self-assessed reading ability and measured reading ability may indicate preclinical visual impairment. Future, larger-scale, C-Read experiments will help determine thresholds for normal and abnormal reading speeds and provide newer, more optimal methods for the early diagnosis of visual impairment.

Supplementary Materials: The following supporting information can be downloaded at https://www.mdpi.com/article/10.3390/jpm13030463/s1: Figure S1: A brief introduction to the C-Read system. (a) There are three different scales, A, B, and C, in C-Read system to assess participants' binocular, right-eye, and left-eye reading ability, respectively. Each scale consists of 16 Chinese sentences, and each sentence consisting of 12 simplified Chinese characters. The length and content of the sentences are carefully selected according to the characteristics of the Chinese language (e.g., sentences with subordinate clauses are not selected, and each sentence contains the same number of simple or complex characters), ensuring that the test tool is adapted to the specific needs of Chinese reading tests. (b) An actual C-Read test: a participant is undergoing a C-Read examination under the supervision of an ophthalmologist. (c) The operating end of C-Read system. The examiner can switch to a different scale for the next test and record the participant's reading time using the C-Read application on the smartphone. Figure S2: The screen of C-Read device. (a) The C-Read system includes a high-definition screen with intelligent display and the ability to synchronize with smartphone application via Bluetooth. The device has a voice recording function and is able to store test data and record patient details. (b) One sentence from another C-Read scale. Specific Chinese sentences are displayed on the screen during the test, and the participant is guided to read them aloud. The font size of the sentences decreases from the top to the bottom. Each time, the screen will only display one sentence. Figure S3: Reading characteristics for left and right eyes for the different sexes, education levels, and myopia levels. (a) The RA for different sexes was statistically significant (n = 191, p = 0.009), as determined by the two-tailed Mann–Whitney test. (b) The MRS for different sexes was not statistically different (n = 191, p = 0.490), as determined by the two-tailed Mann–Whitney test. c) The CPS for different sexes was statistically significant (n = 191, p < 0.001), as determined by the two-tailed Mann–Whitney test. (d) The RA of the three education levels was not significantly different (n = 189, p = 0.252), as determined by the Kruskal–Wallis test. (e) The MRS for the three education levels was statistically significant (n = 189, p = 0.003), as determined by the Kruskal–Wallis test. (f) The CPS for different education levels was not statistically different (n = 189, p = 0.394), as determined by the Kruskal–Wallis test. (g) The RA for different myopia levels was not statistically significant (n = 382 eyes, p = 0.157), as determined by the Kruskal–Wallis test. (h) The MRS for different myopia levels was statistically significant (n = 382 eyes, p = 0.039), as determined by the Kruskal–Wallis test. (i) The CPS for different myopia levels was statistically significant (n = 382 eyes, p < 0.001), as determined by the Kruskal–Wallis test. Abbreviations: RA, reading acuity; MRS, maximum reading speed; CPS, critical print size. Significance: ns, p > 0.05; * p < 0.05; **p < 0.01; *** p < 0.001. Figure S4: Total screen time per day for different genders. The total screen time for different sexes was statistically different (n = 207, p = 0.04), as determined by the Mann–Whitney test. Significance: * p < 0.05. Figure S5: VFQ-25 scores for different genders, education, and myopia. (a) The VFQ-25 scores for different sexes was not statistically different (n = 207, p = 0.22), as determined by a two-tailed Mann–Whitney test. (b) The VFQ-25 scores for different education levels was not statistically different ($n = 189$, $p = 0.24$), as determined by ordinary, one-way ANOVA. (c) The VFQ-25 scores for different myopia levels was not statistically different ($n = 414$ eyes, $p = 0.19$), as determined by ordinary, one-way ANOVA. Abbreviations: VFQ, visual functioning questionnaire. Significance: ns, $p > 0.05$; Table S1. Parameter estimates for MLR model for RA, MRS, and CPS in right, left, and both eyes. Table S2. VFQ-25 sub-scale scores of participants in this study. Table S3. VFQ-25 scores for different genders, education levels, and myopia levels.

Author Contributions: Conceptualization, T.C. and L.S.; data curation, T.C. and B.X.; formal analysis, T.C.; funding acquisition, L.S. and C.Z.; investigation, T.C., B.X. and L.S.; methodology, T.C. and L.S.; software, T.C.; supervision, W.D., X.Q. and J.Y.; writing—original draft, T.C. and T.Y.; writing—review and editing, T.C., T.Y. and L.S. All authors have read and agreed to the published version of the manuscript.

Funding: This study was funded by the Chinese State Natural Science Foundation (Grant No. 81970798), National Science and Technology Key R&D Program (Grant No. 2019YFC0118402), Capital's Funds for Health Improvement and Research of China (Grant No. CFH-2020-2-40911), Young Scientists Fund of the National Natural Science Foundation of China (Grant No. 82201180), and the Peking University Medicine Fund of Fostering Young Scholars' Scientific and Technological Innovation (BMU2022PYB018).

Institutional Review Board Statement: The study was conducted in accordance with the Declaration of Helsinki and approved by the Institutional Review Board of Peking University Third Hospital (IRB00006761-M2022800). The trial was registered with the Chinese Clinical Trial Registry (NCT5673954).

Informed Consent Statement: Informed consent was obtained from all subjects involved in the study.

Data Availability Statement: Data will be made available on request.

Conflicts of Interest: The authors declare no conflict of interest.

References

1. Cieza, A.; Causey, K.; Kamenov, K.; Hanson, S.W.; Chatterji, S.; Vos, T. Global estimates of the need for rehabilitation based on the Global Burden of Disease study 2019: A systematic analysis for the Global Burden of Disease Study 2019. *Lancet* **2021**, *396*, 2006–2017. [CrossRef] [PubMed]
2. Radner, W.; Diendorfer, G.; Kainrath, B.; Kollmitzer, C. The accuracy of reading speed measurement by stopwatch versus measurement with an automated computer program (rad-rd©). *Acta Ophthalmol.* **2017**, *95*, 211–216. [CrossRef] [PubMed]
3. Shah, P.; Schwartz, S.G.; Gartner, S.; Scott, I.U.; Flynn, H.W. Low vision services: A practical guide for the clinician. *Ther. Adv. Ophthalmol.* **2018**, *10*, 2515841418776264. [CrossRef] [PubMed]
4. Kandel, H.; Khadka, J.; Goggin, M.; Pesudovs, K. Impact of refractive error on quality of life: A qualitative study. *Clin. Exp. Ophthalmol.* **2017**, *45*, 677–688. [CrossRef] [PubMed]
5. Elliott, D.B.; Trukolo-Ilic, M.; Strong, J.G.; Pace, R.; Plotkin, A.; Bevers, P. Demographic characteristics of the vision-disabled elderly. *Investig. Ophthalmol. Vis. Sci.* **1997**, *38*, 2566–2575.
6. Hawkins, B.; Miskala, P.; Bass, E.; Bressler, N.; Childs, A.; Mangione, C.; Marsh, M. Submacular Surgery Trials Research Group Surgical removal vs. observation for subfoveal choroidal neovascularization, either associated with the ocular histoplasmosis syndrome or idiopathic: II. Quality-of-life findings from a randomized clinical trial: SST Group H Trial: SST Report No. 10. *Arch Ophthalmol.* **2004**, *122*, 1616–1628. [PubMed]
7. Ghazi, N.G. Bevacizumab for neovascular age-related macular degeneration (ABC trial): Multicenter randomized double-masked study. *Expert Rev. Clin. Pharmacol.* **2010**, *3*, 747–752. [CrossRef]
8. Akutsu, H.; Legge, G.E.; Showalter, M.; Lindstrom, R.L.; Zabel, R.W.; Kirby, V.M. Contrast sensitivity and reading through multifocal intraocular lenses. *Arch. Ophthalmol.* **1992**, *110*, 1076–1080. [CrossRef]
9. Legge, G.E.; Ross, J.A.; Luebker, A.; Lamay, J.M. Psychophysics of reading. VIII. The Minnesota low-vision reading test. *Optom. Vis. Sci.* **1989**, *66*, 843–853. [CrossRef]
10. Mansfield, J.S.; Ahn, S.J.; Legge, G.E.; Luebker, A. A new reading-acuity chart for normal and low vision. In *Noninvasive Assessment of the Visual System*; paper NSuD. 3; Optica Publishing Group: Washington, DC, USA, 1993.
11. Radner, W.; Willinger, U.; Obermayer, W.; Mudrich, C.; Velikay-Parel, M.; Eisenwort, B. A new reading chart for simultaneous determination of reading vision and reading speed. *Klin. Monbl. Augenheilkd.* **1998**, *213*, 174–181. [CrossRef]
12. Radner, W. Standardization of reading charts: A review of recent developments. *Optom. Vis. Sci.* **2019**, *96*, 768–779. [CrossRef]
13. Mansfield, J.S.; Legge, G.E.; Bane, M.C. Psychophysics of reading. XV: Font effects in normal and low vision. *Investig. Ophthalmol. Vis. Sci.* **1996**, *37*, 1492–1501.

14. Han, Q.M.; Cong, L.J.; Yu, C.; Liu, L. Developing a Logarithmic Chinese Reading Acuity Chart. *Optom. Vis. Sci.* **2017**, *94*, 714–724. [CrossRef] [PubMed]
15. Radner, W.; Obermayer, W.; Richter-Mueksch, S.; Willinger, U.; Velikay-Parel, M.; Eisenwort, B. The validity and reliability of short German sentences for measuring reading speed. *Graefes. Arch. Clin. Exp. Ophthalmol.* **2002**, *240*, 461–467. [CrossRef]
16. Hahn, G.A.; Penka, D.; Gehrlich, C.; Messias, A.; Weismann, M.; Hyvärinen, L.; Leinonen, M.; Feely, M.; Rubin, G.; Dauxerre, C.; et al. New standardised texts for assessing reading performance in four European languages. *Br. J. Ophthalmol.* **2006**, *90*, 480–484. [CrossRef] [PubMed]
17. Sultana, A.; Tasnim, S.; Hossain, M.M.; Bhattacharya, S.; Purohit, N. Digital screen time during the COVID-19 pandemic: A public health concern. *F1000Research* **2021**, *10*, 81. [CrossRef]
18. Liu, Z. Reading behavior in the digital environment: Changes in reading behavior over the past ten years. *J. Doc.* **2005**, *61*, 700–712. [CrossRef]
19. Legge, G.E. Reading digital with low vision. *Visible Lang.* **2016**, *50*, 102.
20. Kingsnorth, A.; Wolffsohn, J.S. Mobile app reading speed test. *Br. J. Ophthalmol.* **2015**, *99*, 536–539. [CrossRef]
21. Calabrèse, A.; To, L.; He, Y.; Berkholtz, E.; Rafian, P.; Legge, G.E. Comparing performance on the MNREAD iPad application with the MNREAD acuity chart. *J. Vis.* **2018**, *18*, 8. [CrossRef]
22. Calabrese, A.; Gamam, S.; Mansfield, J.S.; Legge, G.E. Implementing the MNREAD Reading Acuity Test on an ipad3. *READING* **2014**, *200*, 300.
23. Murro, V.; Sodi, A.; Giacomelli, G.; Mucciolo, D.P.; Pennino, M.; Virgili, G.; Rizzo, S. Reading Ability and Quality of Life in Stargardt Disease. *Eur. J. Ophthalmol.* **2017**, *27*, 740–745. [CrossRef] [PubMed]
24. Moher, D.; Hopewell, S.; Schulz, K.F.; Montori, V.; Gøtzsche, P.C.; Devereaux, P.J.; Elbourne, D.; Egger, M.; Altman, D.G. CONSORT 2010 explanation and elaboration: Updated guidelines for reporting parallel group randomised trials. *BMJ* **2010**, *340*, c869. [CrossRef]
25. Mangione, C.M.; Lee, P.P.; Gutierrez, P.R.; Spritzer, K.; Berry, S.; Hays, R.D. Development of the 25-item National Eye Institute Visual Function Questionnaire. *Arch. Ophthalmol.* **2001**, *119*, 1050–1058. [PubMed]
26. Broman, A.T.; Munoz, B.; West, S.K.; Rodriguez, J.; Sanchez, R.; Snyder, R.; Klein, R. Psychometric properties of the 25-item NEI-VFQ in a Hispanic population: Proyecto VER. *Investig. Ophthalmol. Vis. Sci.* **2001**, *42*, 606–613.
27. Globe, D.; Varma, R.; Azen, S.P.; Paz, S.; Yu, E.; Preston-Martin, S. Psychometric performance of the NEI VFQ-25 in visually normal Latinos: The Los Angeles Latino Eye Study. *Investig. Ophthalmol. Vis. Sci.* **2003**, *44*, 1470–1478. [CrossRef]
28. Suzukamo, Y.; Oshika, T.; Yuzawa, M.; Tokuda, Y.; Tomidokoro, A.; Oki, K.; Mangione, C.M.; Green, J.; Fukuhara, S. Psychometric properties of the 25-item National Eye Institute Visual Function Questionnaire (NEI VFQ-25), Japanese version. *Health Qual. Life Outcomes* **2005**, *3*, 65. [CrossRef]
29. Labiris, G.; Katsanos, A.; Fanariotis, M.; Tsirouki, T.; Pefkianaki, M.; Chatzoulis, D.; Tsironi, E. Psychometric properties of the Greek version of the NEI-VFQ 25. *BMC Ophthalmol.* **2008**, *8*, 4. [CrossRef]
30. Chan, C.W.; Wong, D.; Lam, C.L.; McGhee, S.; Lai, W.W. Development of a Chinese version of the National Eye Institute Visual Function Questionnaire (CHI-VFQ-25) as a tool to study patients with eye diseases in Hong Kong. *Br. J. Ophthalmol.* **2009**, *93*, 1431–1436. [CrossRef]
31. Grosvenor, T. A review and a suggested classification system for myopia on the basis of age-related prevalence and age of onset. *Am. J. Optom. Physiol. Opt.* **1987**, *64*, 545–554. [CrossRef]
32. Rubin, G.S. Measuring reading performance. *Vis. Res.* **2013**, *90*, 43–51. [CrossRef] [PubMed]
33. Lovie-Kitchin, J.E.; Bowers, A.R.; Woods, R.L. Oral and silent reading performance with macular degeneration. *Ophthalmic Physiol. Opt.* **2000**, *20*, 360–370. [CrossRef] [PubMed]
34. Runge, P.E. Eduard Jaeger's Test-Types (Schrift-Scalen) and the historical development of vision tests. *Trans. Am. Ophthalmol. Soc.* **2000**, *98*, 375–438. [PubMed]
35. Trauzettel-Klosinski, S.; Dietz, K.; Group, I.S. Standardized assessment of reading performance: The new international reading speed texts IReST. *Investig. Ophthalmol. Vis. Sci.* **2012**, *53*, 5452–5461. [CrossRef]
36. Cheung, J.P.; Liu, D.S.; Lam, C.C.; Cheong, A.M. Development and validation of a new Chinese reading chart for children. *Ophthalmic Physiol. Opt.* **2015**, *35*, 514–521. [CrossRef]
37. Zhang, J.Y.; Zhang, T.; Xue, F.; Liu, L.; Yu, C. Legibility variations of Chinese characters and implications for visual acuity measurement in Chinese reading population. *Investig. Ophthalmol. Vis. Sci.* **2007**, *48*, 2383–2390. [CrossRef]
38. West, S.K.; Rubin, G.S.; Munoz, B.; Abraham, D.; Fried, L.P.; The Salisbury Eye Evaluation Project T. Assessing Functional Status: Correlation Between Performance on Tasks Conducted in a Clinic Setting and Performance on the Same Task Conducted at Home. *J. Gerontol. Ser. A* **1997**, *52A*, M209–M217. [CrossRef]
39. Fried, L.P.; Herdman, S.J.; Kuhn, K.E.; Rubin, G.; Turano, K. Preclinical disability: Hypotheses about the bottom of the iceberg. *J. Aging Health* **1991**, *3*, 285–300. [CrossRef]
40. Pan, C.W.; Ramamurthy, D.; Saw, S.M. Worldwide prevalence and risk factors for myopia. *Ophthalmic Physiol. Opt.* **2012**, *32*, 3–16. [CrossRef]
41. Huang, L.; Kawasaki, H.; Liu, Y.; Wang, Z. The prevalence of myopia and the factors associated with it among university students in Nanjing: A cross-sectional study. *Medicine* **2019**, *98*, e14777. [CrossRef]

42. Hu, Y.; Zhao, F.; Ding, X.; Zhang, S.; Li, Z.; Guo, Y.; Feng, Z.; Tang, X.; Li, Q.; Guo, L.; et al. Rates of Myopia Development in Young Chinese Schoolchildren During the Outbreak of COVID-19. *JAMA Ophthalmol.* **2021**, *139*, 1115–1121. [CrossRef] [PubMed]
43. Balhara, Y.P.S.; Bhargava, R. Screen time and COVID-19: Observations from among the college students in India. *J. Behav. Addict* **2022**, *11*, 182.
44. Seresirikachorn, K.; Thiamthat, W.; Sriyuttagrai, W.; Soonthornworasiri, N.; Singhanetr, P.; Yudtanahiran, N.; Theeramunkong, T. Effects of digital devices and online learning on computer vision syndrome in students during the COVID-19 era: An online questionnaire study. *BMJ Paediatr. Open* **2022**, *6*, e001429. [CrossRef] [PubMed]
45. Guo, Y.F.; Liao, M.Q.; Cai, W.L.; Yu, X.X.; Li, S.N.; Ke, X.Y.; Tan, S.X.; Luo, Z.Y.; Cui, Y.F.; Wang, Q.; et al. Physical activity, screen exposure and sleep among students during the pandemic of COVID-19. *Sci. Rep.* **2021**, *11*, 8529. [CrossRef] [PubMed]
46. Lissak, G. Adverse physiological and psychological effects of screen time on children and adolescents: Literature review and case study. *Environ. Res.* **2018**, *164*, 149–157. [CrossRef]
47. Wong, C.W.; Tsai, A.; Jonas, J.B.; Ohno-Matsui, K.; Chen, J.; Ang, M.; Ting, D.S.W. Digital Screen Time During the COVID-19 Pandemic: Risk for a Further Myopia Boom? *Am. J. Ophthalmol.* **2021**, *223*, 333–337. [CrossRef] [PubMed]
48. Mu, J.; Zhong, H.; Liu, M.; Jiang, M.; Shuai, X.; Chen, Y.; Long, W.; Zhang, S. Trends in Myopia Development Among Primary and Secondary School Students During the COVID-19 Pandemic: A Large-Scale Cross-Sectional Study. *Front. Public Health* **2022**, *10*, 859285. [CrossRef]
49. Liu, J.; Chen, Q.; Dang, J. Examining risk factors related to digital learning and social isolation: Youth visual acuity in COVID-19 pandemic. *J. Glob. Health.* **2021**, *11*, 05020. [CrossRef]
50. Calabrèse, A.; Cheong, A.M.; Cheung, S.H.; He, Y.; Kwon, M.; Mansfield, J.S.; Subramanian, A.; Yu, D.; Legge, G.E. Baseline MNREAD Measures for Normally Sighted Subjects From Childhood to Old Age. *Investig. Ophthalmol. Vis. Sci.* **2016**, *57*, 3836–3843. [CrossRef]
51. Chan, C.W.; Wong, J.C.; Chan, K.S.; Wong, W.K.; Tam, K.C.; Chau, P.S. Evaluation of quality of life in patients with cataract in Hong Kong. *J. Cataract. Refract. Surg.* **2003**, *29*, 1753–1760.
52. Zhu, M.; Yu, J.; Zhang, J.; Yan, Q.; Liu, Y. Evaluating vision-related quality of life in preoperative age-related cataract patients and analyzing its influencing factors in China: A cross-sectional study. *BMC Ophthalmol.* **2015**, *15*, 160. [CrossRef] [PubMed]
53. Hernandez Trillo, A.; Dickinson, C.M. The impact of visual and nonvisual factors on quality of life and adaptation in adults with visual impairment. *Investig. Ophthalmol. Vis. Sci.* **2012**, *53*, 4234–4241. [CrossRef] [PubMed]

Journal of *Personalized Medicine*

MDPI

Article

A Modified Technique for Preventing Lens–Iris Diaphragm Retropulsion Syndrome in Vitrectomized Eyes during Phacoemulsification

Zhiyi Wu [1], Tian He [2], Zhitao Su [1], Ye Liu [1], Jingliang He [1] and Yanan Huo [1,*]

1 Eye Center, The Second Affiliated Hospital, Zhejiang University School of Medicine, Hangzhou 310010, China
2 Department of Ophthalmology, The Children's Hospital of Hangzhou, Hangzhou 310010, China
* Correspondence: 3309035@zju.edu.cn; Tel.: +86-0571-8778-3897

Abstract: Background: Lens–iris diaphragm retropulsion syndrome (LIDRS) is common in vitrectomized or high myopic eyes during phacoemulsification. We evaluated the results of a modified technique for cataract treatment using phacoemulsification in vitrectomized eyes. Methods: In this retrospective study, we enrolled thirty-four vitrectomized eyes treated with modified phacoemulsification (Modified Group) and nineteen vitrectomized eyes treated with routine phacoemulsification (Control Group). The modified technique comprised irrigation with a balanced salt solution underneath the pupil before phacoemulsification instrument entry, lens implantation and stromal hydration to stabilize the anterior chamber and equilibrate the pressure between the anterior chamber and posterior cavity. Results: We compared the incidences of intra and postoperative complications and visual outcomes between modified and routine phacoemulsification. Pain, LIDRS and difficulty in stromal hydration were significantly more common in the Control Group than in the Modified Group ($p < 0.05$). There were no significant differences in the rates of posterior capsular rupture, iris trauma, lens dislocation, or posterior capsular opacification between the Modified and Control Groups ($p > 0.05$). However, there was no significant difference in visual acuity between the groups ($p > 0.05$). Complications such as loss of nuclear fragments into the vitreous cavity, cystoid macular edema, retina redetachment, suprachoroidal hemorrhage and vitreous hemorrhage did not occur either intra or postoperatively in any of our patients. Conclusions: Our modified technique prevents LIDRS and complications arising during cataract surgery in vitrectomized eyes. Aside from this, the results of modified and routine phacoemulsification are similar in vitrectomized eyes.

Keywords: modified technique; phacoemulsification; vitrectomized eyes; lens–iris diaphragm retropulsion

Citation: Wu, Z.; He, T.; Su, Z.; Liu, Y.; He, J.; Huo, Y. A Modified Technique for Preventing Lens–Iris Diaphragm Retropulsion Syndrome in Vitrectomized Eyes during Phacoemulsification. *J. Pers. Med.* **2023**, *13*, 418. https://doi.org/10.3390/jpm13030418

Academic Editors: Kai Jin and Chun Zhang

Received: 5 December 2022
Revised: 4 February 2023
Accepted: 22 February 2023
Published: 26 February 2023

1. Introduction

A cataract is an eye disease that involves the opacification of the crystalline lens of the eye or its envelope. There are many known causes of cataracts, including the natural aging process, nutritional disorders, metabolic abnormalities such as diabetes, chronic ocular inflammation and certain injuries. Intraocular surgery is the gold standard for cataract surgery. But it can format or accelerate cataracts, especially pars plana vitrectomy (PPV), which is a microsurgical technique to treat certain disorders affecting the posterior segment of the eyes. During vitrectomy surgery, three small incisions are made in the eye in order to place the following instruments: a fiberoptic light source to illuminate the inside of the eye, a vitreous cutter, and an infusion cannula to maintain proper intraocular pressure during the surgery. Advances in PPV surgical techniques and instrumentation have revolutionized the treatment of posterior segment disorders. However, there remain some surgical risks of significant vision loss, including retinal detachment, corneal endothelial decompensation and cataract formation or progression in phakic eyes. Nuclear sclerotic cataract development is the most frequent complication after pars plana vitrectomy (PPV) in the phakic eye [1,2]. However, phacoemulsification is a challenge in the vitrectomized eye because of the lack of vitreous support, the unstable anterior chamber depth and the density of the nuclear cataract. In addition, intraoperative complications such as intraoperative ocular pain and lens dislocation can also increase the difficulty of surgical procedures. Additionally, the risk and incidence of complications are higher in cataract surgery after a previous PPV than in non-PPV eyes. Hence, phacoemulsification in the vitrectomized eye is associated with higher rates of intra and postoperative complications [3–8].

Lens–iris diaphragm retropulsion syndrome (LIDRS) was first described in 1992 by Zauberman and further named by Wilbrandt and Wilbrandt in 1994 [9–19]. The incidence rate of LIDRS in vitrectomized eyes during phacoemulsification widely varies, ranging from 4.5% to 100% [11,12]. The syndrome is characterized by the anterior chamber (AC) deepening, followed by pupil dilation and a typical concave iris configuration. During cataract surgery, as the initial corneal incision is made, fluid is lost from both the AC and the vitreous cavity, resulting in the loss of AC and vitreous body volumes. When phacoemulsification or irrigation/aspiration (I/A) probes are inserted, the irrigation causes significant differences in the pressure between the anterior and posterior compartments. The AC deepens, and the iris bows posterior to the lens, blocking fluid passage from the AC. The surgeon must adjust the operative plane by positioning the instruments deeper, which may deform the incision and compromise performance. During phacoemulsification or cortical aspiration, the probe is positioned posterior to the iris plane, resulting in changes in fluid dynamics. Fluid may enter the vitreous cavity through zonular defects, increasing posterior cavity pressure and causing shallowing of the AC and miosis. IDS can lead to complications, such as posterior capsular rupture (PCR), iris trauma, expulsive choroidal hemorrhage and choroidal detachment.

The literature on LIDRS prevention during cataract surgery in vitrectomized eyes is scarce [6]. To minimize LIDRS and LIDRS-related complications, we modified the technique by irrigating a balanced salt solution (BSS) into the vitreous cavity through a syringe with a bent, blunt-tipped needle. This technique stabilized the AC intraoperatively, preventing abrupt excursions of the iris–lens diaphragm and making emulsification, cortical aspiration, intraocular lens (IOL) implantation and stromal hydration safer.

In this retrospective study, we compared the intra and postoperative complications of the modified (Modified Group) and routine (Control Group) phacoemulsification surgeries in eyes after 23-gauge PPV.

2. Materials and Methods

2.1. Participants

We retrospectively reviewed the medical records of 59 patients (62 eyes) who underwent consecutive phacoemulsification and IOL implantation after a previous 23-gauge three-port PPV surgery between 12 January 2015 and 31 December 2016 in the Eye Center of the Second Affiliated Hospital of Zhejiang University School of Medicine. Patients with in situ silicone oil were excluded from the study. This study followed the tenets of the *Declaration of Helsinki*. The Ethics Committee of the Second Affiliated Hospital of Zhejiang University School of Medicine approved this study (No. 2015-003).

Data were gathered on age, sex, indications for PPV, indications of PPV, preoperative evaluations, intraoperative observations and complications. The patients were followed-up postoperatively on day 1, as well as 1, 2, 4, 8, 12 and 24 weeks after their cataract surgery. Visual acuity and intraocular pressure assessments and slit-lamp examinations were performed, and any postoperative complications were noted. Neodymium-yttrium-aluminum-garnet (Nd: YAG) laser posterior capsulotomy was performed for residual posterior capsular opacification.

2.2. Surgical Techniques

All vitrectomy and cataract surgeries were conducted by a single experienced surgeon using the associate vitrectomy and phacoemulsification machine (Stellaris PC; Bausch +

Lomb: Rochester, NY, USA). All the patients underwent cataract surgery under topical anesthesia (proparacaine hydrochloride 0.5%).

In the Control Group, a side port corneal incision was created with a blade initially. A small amount of viscoelastic was then injected into the anterior chamber before the 2 mm superior corneal incision was made. A continuous curvilinear capsulorrhexis was made under viscoelastic in all eyes. Hydrodissection was performed using a BSS supplemented with adrenaline. The nucleus was chopped using the "phaco-chop" or "stop-and-chop" methods. A 30° phacoemulsification probe was used for all the patients. Cortical clean-up was performed using an I/A probe. A foldable IOL (CT ASPHINA 509M; Carl Zeiss Meditec: Jena, Germany/iSert® 250; Hoya Surgical Optics Inc.: Chino Hills, CA, USA) was implanted into the capsular bag. Any residual viscoelastic material was completely removed from the AC and behind the IOL with an I/A probe. The stromal hydration of the side port and main incision was performed using the BSS. At the end of the procedure, a 0.1% TobraDex® ointment (Alcon Laboratories, Inc.: Fort Worth, TX, USA) was administered.

The main steps of the modified technique, including phacoemulsification, I/A, IOL implantation and stromal hydration, were the same as those of routine cataract surgery. However, to stabilize the AC, we irrigated the BSS underneath the pupil using a syringe with a bent, blunt-tipped needle for a few seconds, which allowed the fluid to enter the vitreous cavity (Figure 1). This irrigation was performed before phacoemulsification, I/A probe entry, IOL insertion and stromal hydration to enable pressure equilibration between the anterior and posterior cavities, to prevent abrupt excursions of the iris–lens diaphragm and to facilitate sculpting and nuclear fragmentation (Figure 2).

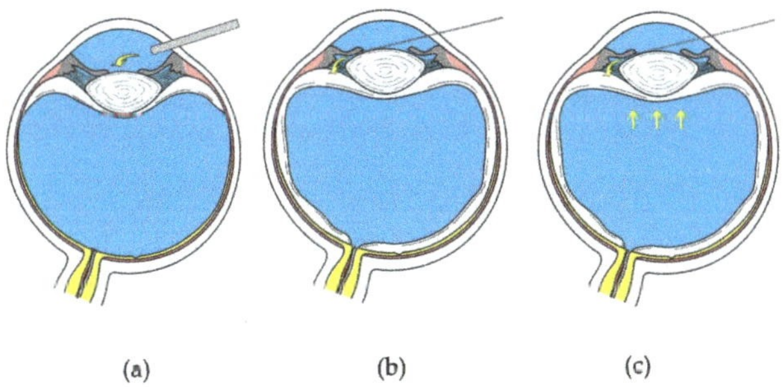

Figure 1. Images demonstrating intraocular fluidics in vitrectomized eyes before and after the modified technique. (**a**) As the irrigating phacoemulsification probe enters the anterior chamber, the iris-lens diaphragm is displaced posteriorly, creating a relative pupillary block. (**b**) Lens–iris diaphragm retropulsion syndrome controlled by lifting the iris with the needle and irrigating a balanced salt solution underneath the iris, allowing flow of fluid into the vitreous cavity. (**c**) This technique stabilizes the iris-lens diaphragm as the pressure equilibrates.

The surgeries were recorded using a video system and analyzed for both groups. The settings for phacoemulsification (Stellaris PC) were as follows: phacoemulsification power, 0–50% (depending on the grade of the nucleus), and vacuum limit, 350 mmHg. The bottle height was 90 cm above the patient's head.

2.3. Statistical Analysis

SPSS 23.0 software (IBM: Armonk, New York, NY, USA) was used for all statistical analyses. Data were presented as the mean ± standard deviation or as n (%) for categorical variables. We used Student's t-test for normally distributed variables, the Kruskal–Wallis test for non-parametric variables, and the chi-squared or Fisher's exact tests, as indicated for the analyses of categorical variables. Snellen's best-corrected visual acuity measurements were converted to the logarithm of the minimum angle of resolution (logMAR) equivalents for the purpose of data analysis. A p-value of <0.05 was considered statistically significant.

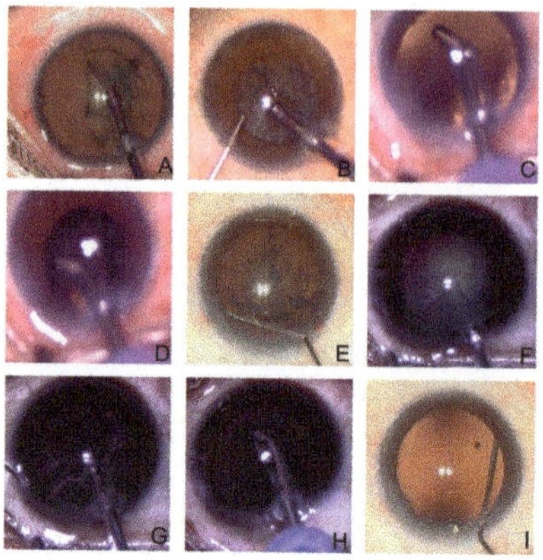

Figure 2. Photographs demonstrating our surgical technique to manage infusion deviation syndrome. (**A**) When the phacoemulsification probe is first inserted, the anterior chamber (AC) deepens, and pupil size increases in Control Group. (**B**) The changes in fluid dynamics cause shallowing of the AC, with miosis following immediately during emulsification in the Control Group. (**C**,**D**) The same phenomena (infusion deviation syndrome) occur during cortical aspiration. (**E**) Before emulsification, a BSS is irrigated underneath the pupil to stabilize the AC in the Modified Group. (**F**,**G**) With the modified irrigation technique, the AC depth remains stable during emulsification procedures in the Modified Group. (**H**) The AC depth remains stable during cortical aspiration in the Modified Group. (**I**) The modified technique performed before IOL insertion.

3. Results

This retrospective study enrolled 59 patients (62 eyes). Seven patients (nine eyes) with in situ silicone oil were excluded from this study. The mean age of the patients in the Modified Group was 64.03 ± 13.12 years, whereas that of patients in the Control Group was 57 ± 12.31 years ($p > 0.05$). There were twenty-one male and thirteen female patients in the Modified Group and thirteen male and six female patients (19 eyes) in the Control Group ($p > 0.05$). The interval between PPV and phacoemulsification was not significantly different between the Modified (8.39 ± 4.7 months) and Control (9.9 ± 5.22 months) Groups.

Table 1 summarizes the indication for PPV. The indications for PPV in the Modified Group were retinal detachment in 18/34 eyes (52.9%), macular hole in 5/34 eyes (14.7%), proliferative diabetic retinopathy in 5/34 eyes (14.7%), epiretinal membrane in 4/34 eyes (11.8%) and retinal vein occlusion in 2/34 eyes (5.9%). In contrast, in the Control Group, the indications for PPV were retinal detachment in 8/19 eyes (42.1%), a macular hole in 5/19 eyes (26.3%), proliferative diabetic retinopathy in 3/19 eyes (15.8%), retinal vein occlusion in 2/19 eyes (10.5%) and epiretinal membrane in 1/19 eyes (5.3%; Table 1). The indications for PPV were not significantly different between the Modified Group and Control Group (all $p > 0.05$).

Table 1. Indications for pars plana vitrectomy (PPV) in the Modified and Control Groups.

Indication for PPV	Modified Group (n = 34)	Total Number of Eyes (n = 53) Control Group (n = 19)	p Value
Retinal detachment	18 (52.9%)	8 (42.1%)	0.45
Macular hole	5 (14.7%)	5 (26.3%)	0.3
Proliferative diabetic retinophathy	5 (14.7%)	3 (15.8%)	0.922
itreous hemorhage	4 (11.8%)	2 (10.5%)	0.89
piretinal membrane	2 (5.9%)	1 (5.3%)	0.93

Table 1 was analyzed using chi-square tests, with continuity correction and Fisher's Exact Test.

Table 2 summarizes the intraoperative observations and complications encountered. Not all vitrectomized eyes developed LIDRS in our study. Characteristically, the anterior chamber depth appeared abnormal as soon as irrigation commenced. The iris-lens diaphragm bowed posteriorly, causing the anterior chamber to deepen excessively and the pupil to dilate widely. During nuclear sculpting, the deepening of the abnormal anterior chamber necessitated steeper angulation of the phacoemulsification probe, and the nucleus was also noted to be more mobile than usual. Intraoperatively, LIDRS was noted in 2/34 eyes (5.9%) in the Modified Group and in 8/19 eyes (42.1%) in the Control Group ($p < 0.05$; Table 2). Patients with 11/19 eyes (57.9%) in the Control Group complained of sudden pain (in the range of 2–3 out of 10 on the numerical rating scale) when instruments entered the AC, whereas none of the 34 patients in the Modified Group felt pain ($p < 0.05$). In the Control Group, 1/19 eyes (5.3%) had PCR, and the IOL was placed in the ciliary sulcus. Additionally, in the Control Group, 2/19 eyes (10.5%) developed iris trauma during aspiration of the cortex and viscoelastic material. However, IOL dislocation occurred in only 1/34 eyes (2.9%) in the Modified Groupand was replaced in the capsular bag immediately. Difficulty in stromal hydration was observed in 4/34 eyes (11.8%) in the Modified Group and 7/19 eyes (36.8%) in the Control Group ($p < 0.05$). Cataract surgery was completed in all cases, in both the Modified Group and the Control Group.

Table 2. Intraoperative and postoperative observations and complications encountered.

Complication	Modified Group (n = 34)	Total Number of Eyes (n = 53) Control Group (n = 19)	p Value
Intraoperative			
LIDRS	2 (5.9%)	8 (42.1%)	0.001 *
Pain	0 (0%)	11 (57.9%)	<0.001 *
Posterior capsular rupture	0 (0%)	1 (5.3%)	0.177
Iris trauma	0 (0%)	2 (10.5%)	0.054
Dislocation of IOL	1 (2.9%)	0 (0%)	0.45
Difficulty in stromal hydration	4 (11.8%)	7 (36.8%)	0.03 *
Postoperative			
PCO requiring Nd: YAG laser capsulotomy	9 (26.5%)	5 (26.3%)	0.99

Table 2 were analyzed by chi-square tests, with continuity correction and Fisher's Exact Test. * $p < 0.05$, statistically significant.

No complications, such as loss of nuclear fragments into the vitreous cavity, cystoid macular edema, retinal redetachment, suprachoroidal hemorrhage, or vitreous hemorrhage, occurred either intra or postoperatively in any of the patients. Posterior capsular opacification was evident in 9/34 eyes (26.5%) in the Modified Group and in 5/19 eyes (26.3%) in the Control Group ($p = 0.99$); this was successfully removed using the Nd: YAG laser. No patients in either group required any surgical intervention in the 24-week follow-up period (Table 2).

The final visual outcomes were dictated by the nature of the retinal pathology present at the time of the initial vitrectomy procedure. The mean preoperative best-corrected visual acuity of the Modified Group was 1.11 ± 0.46 logMAR units, and that of the Control Group was 1.13 ± 0.52 logMAR units. Both improved significantly at 24 weeks after surgery, to 0.58± 0.35 logMAR units in the Modified Group and 0.59 ± 0.43 logMAR units in the Control Group (both $p < 0.005$). The final visual acuity was similar between the groups ($p > 0.05$). External segment, ocular motility, pupillary function and intraocular pressure were within normal limits in both groups.

4. Discussion

PPV was first developed by Machemer in 1971. It is an effective, small-gauge, safe surgery that is essential in the treatment of a variety of posterior segment pathologies, including retinal detachment, macular hole, proliferative diabetic retinopathy, vitreous hemorrhage due to diabetic retinopathy or vein occlusion, preretinal membrane and endophthalmitis. However, performing a vitrectomy can induce cataracts, particularly with the use of intraocular gas, even in young patients. Cataracts eventually occur in almost all eyes after PPV [13]. The causative factors of cataract formation or acceleration after PPV have been linked with the use of intraocular gas, oxidation of lens protein, light toxicity, length of operative time and oxygen tension within the eye. In non-vitrectomized eyes, the vitreous body (especially the vitreous base) limits the flow of fluid from the posterior chamber into the vitreous cavity, preventing changes in volume and pressure in both the AC and posterior segment. However, phacoemulsification in vitrectomized eyes is more technically challenging than that in nonvitrectomized eyes [14]. The primary reason for this is the loss of vitreous counterpressure in vitrectomized eyes. Some vitrectomized eyes also have localized zonular weaknesses caused by loss of the vitreous scaffold, stretching of the zonules by expansile gas or oil, or damage to the zonular apparatus during vitrectomy [15]. This may lead to faster and easier fluid exchange between the AC and posterior cavity. Extremely stretched zonules can be easy to break, causing lens dislocation. Additionally, strong fluctuations in the AC or the iris–capsular bag diaphragm may cause patients pain and trigger unexpected abrupt agitation, increasing the difficulty of the surgery [16]. The nucleus tends to be harder than in age-related nuclear sclerosis, requiring longer phacoemulsification time during the procedure. Together, the unstable posterior capsule and zonules, extended operative time and increased pain experienced by the patients increase the likelihood of complications such as expulsive choroidal hemorrhage or choroidal detachment. With the increasing use of vitrectomy in the treatment of various posterior segment disorders, we expect to see an increase in the number of such cataracts being referred to general ophthalmologists and anterior segment surgeons. Unfortunately, most complications are unpredictable. Specific surgical experience and skills related to the management of complications during cataract surgery in vitrectomized eyes are required.

Many studies have reported that phacoemulsification is surgically more challenging in vitrectomized eyes than in nonvitrectomized eyes because various anatomic changes within the eye confer a higher risk of complications. In 1992, Zauberman [8] first described the phenomenon of AC deepening, excessive pupil dilation and a concave shape of the iris during phacoemulsification. Wilbrandt and Wilbrant further studied this syndrome and named it LIDRS in 1994 [7]. LIDRS are more likely to happen in eyes that have had multiple or extensive PPV for diabetic proliferative retinopathy and retinal detachment. However, less LIDRS or abnormally deep AC was evident in eyes that had undergone a limited "core vitrectomy", such as for a macular hole or epiretinal membrane. In our study, of the ten patients noted to develop LIDRS, eight had undergone thorough PPV for retinal detachment or diabetic proliferative retinopathy. These eight patients previously had thorough vitreous removal through peripheral indentation and trimming of the vitreous base in order to relieve anterior vitreous traction. These procedures may have caused structural damage in the vitreous base region, resulting in abnormal laxity of the zonules. Szijarto et al. [17] observed a deep or fluctuating AC in 93% of vitrectomized eyes, implying that the occurrence of LIDRS is related to the loss of the vitreous body, especially the vitreous base. Other studies have reported that the rate of LIDRS-related complications, such as PCR during cataract surgery in vitrectomized eyes, ranges from 0 to 11.4% [6,7,17–23]. The rate of dropped nuclei ranges from 0 to 4.5% [6,7,17–24], while the rate of zonular dialyses ranges from 0 to 5% [6,7,17–19,24], and the rate of iris trauma ranges from 0 to 0.2% [20,21,24]. The rate of posterior capsular opacification requiring Nd: YAG laser capsulotomy after cataract surgery reportedly ranges from 2.2 to 44% in vitrectomized eyes, depending on the follow-up period [6,17–19,24]. The rate of retinal detachment in the early postoperative period after cataract surgery in vitrectomized eyes ranges from 1.2 to 6% [17–19,24]. The rate of decentration and dislocation of the IOL is around 2 to 2.9% [18,22], whilst the rate of hypotony with choroidal effusion ranges from 0 to 0.6% [18,20,21], and the rate of vitreous hemorrhage ranges from 0.6 to 6% [18,19]. Valesová L et al. reported in 2004 that the incidence of intraoperative complications in the posterior perfusion cataract surgery was slightly higher than in the standard cataract surgery group; there were no special complications in the standard cataract surgery group. Furthermore, the safety of the two surgical methods was consistent [25]. In this study, our findings were significantly different from the study by Valesová L et al. in 2004, as the method in our study differs from theirs. Our method is simple, fast, safe, non-invasive and does not require additional equipment. However, their study used an invasive method to create a new perfusion hole in the eye, which would increase the eyeball damage, the length of the operation and the back pressure, resulting in other complications. In addition, their study showed that their invasive approach does not reduce the risk of surgery.

In contrast, we experienced significantly fewer complications during cataract surgery using the modified technique. Pain upon the entry of irrigation into the AC did not occur in the Modified Group; however it was reported by 57.9% of the Control Group ($p < 0.05$). The rates of LIDRS and iris trauma were also significantly lower in the Modified Group than in the Control Group (both $p < 0.05$).

Immediately closing corneal incisions after surgery is important for preventing postoperative complications such as hypotony, choroidal effusion and endophthalmitis. However, stromal hydration can be hindered by ocular hypotony during surgery in vitrectomized eyes. Sachdev et al. [20] reported a rate of early postoperative hypotony and serous choroidal detachment of 1.3% after cataract surgery in vitrectomized eyes. Other authors have reported the use of 10/0 sutures to seal the corneal incision [18]. However, in our study, irrigation with a BSS before sealing the incisions seemed sufficient for solving this problem and preventing related complications. The rate of difficulty in sealing the corneal incision was significantly lower in the Modified Group than in the Control Group ($p < 0.05$).

One patient (2.9%) in the Modified Group experienced IOL dislocation caused by excessive irrigation during stromal hydration. The IOL was repositioned, and relatively good visual performance was attained without further treatment.

Patients who develop cataracts after PPV surgery may undergo a phacoemulsification cataract surgery. Although visual acuity in a normal eye typically improves after cataract surgery, the visual prognosis after surgery for post vitrectomy cataract may be uncertain. Visual acuity and other outcomes after phacoemulsification cataract surgery in eyes undergoing vitrectomy are dependent on multiple factors, although primarily on the retinal condition and the avoidance of complications during cataract surgery. In our experience, the patients who had undergone PPV for macula-on retinal detachment or a macular hole experienced a better improvement in visual acuity after cataract surgery. The patients who had undergone PPV for macula-off retinal detachment or proliferative diabetic retinopathy experienced less visual improvement. There were no severe complications, such as dropped nuclei, expulsive choroidal hemorrhage or choroidal detachment, in the present study. The number of eyes that received Nd: YAG laser treatment after cataract surgery did not differ between the two groups in this study; this confirms the safety of the modified procedure.

The timing of irrigation in our modified technique is important. As both the AC and vitreous body fluid are continually lost from the corneal incision, we balanced the pressure between the AC and posterior segment by irrigation of a BSS underneath the iris at four time points:

(1) Before the first entry of the phacoemulsification probe;
(2) Before the first entry of the I/A probe;
(3) Before the insertion of the IOL; and
(4) Before the hydration of the stromal incision.

This modified irrigation regimen allows fluid to enter the posterior segment, resulting in pressure equilibration. Using the above steps not only made operating on these eyes safer, since the phaco handpiece could be held in a normal position, but it also greatly enhanced the patient's comfort. As shown in Table 2, this irrigation significantly decreased the incidences of pain, LIDRS, PCR and difficulty in stromal hydration (all $p < 0.05$).

In our study, all of the patients had phacoemulsification cataract surgery through a superior corneal incision instead of a scleral tunnel. In our opinion, it is preferable to have a steeper angulation of the phacoemulsification probe when operating on vitrectomized eyes. Using a corneal incision also avoids conjunctival scarring or postoperative infection resulting from occult filtration.

In our experience, LIDRS does not only occur in phakic eyes after PPV; it also occurs in eyes with high myopia as a result of synchysis, greater AC and axial lengths, a floppy posterior capsule and zonular laxity. High myopia eyes with elongated stretched zonular fibers are more prone to develop LIDRS during phacoemulsification cataract surgery. Additional techniques can be used in vitrectomized and high myopic eyes to minimize IDS, such as reducing the height of the liquid bottle to about 90 cm, using a low-flow rate and vacuum limit, and using a finger to press the corneal incision. A longer, better self-sealing corneal incision and a shorter interval between each step may decrease fluid loss and intraocular pressure fluctuation, meaning that the AC may remain watertight.

Other authors have advocated different solutions for stabilizing the AC, such as forming the AC with viscoelastic material during the routine phacoemulsification procedure [2]. An AC maintainer and an irrigating chopper have also been reported to prevent AC fluctuation [26,27]; however, an AC maintainer requires an additional corneal incision. The use of an irrigating chopper in microincisional cataract surgery in tandem with cold phacoemulsification technology has been reported; however, the issue of wound burns persists because of the "naked" phacoemulsification needle [3,6,28]. Joshi [29] modified the sleeve of a phacoemulsification probe to increase fluid flow and deepen the capsular bag, with the aim of decreasing the fluctuation in the AC. However, both prospective and retrospective comparative studies on the prevention of LIDRS in vitrectomized eyes after cataract surgery are lacking [7]. Our study had certain limitations. There are significant astigmatic changes during the early postoperative period and posterior capsular transparency changes during the late postoperative period. Continued follow-ups of the patients are necessary to monitor the long-term refractive stability and visual acuity of these procedures.

5. Conclusions

In summary, our time-saving technique has demonstrated good surgical results in this retrospective study. This simple technique increases fluid flow into the vitreous cavity, resulting in pressure equilibration and a reduced risk of complications without using additional instruments during routine cataract surgery. The rate of LIDRS and related complications were relatively low compared with the Control Groupand the findings of previous studies. Therefore, we recommend considering this approach in patients with a history of PPV.

Author Contributions: Conceptualization: Z.W. and Y.H.; Data curation: Z.S. and J.H.; Formal analysis: Z.S., T.H. and Y.L.; Investigation: Y.L.; Methodology: Z.W. and Y.H.; Software: Z.S. and J.H.; Writing—original draft: Z.W.; Writing—review & editing: T.H., Y.L., J.H. and Y.H. All authors have read and agreed to the published version of the manuscript.

Funding: This work was supported by the Zhejiang Provincial Natural Science Foundation (LY20H 120009), the National Natural Science Foundation of China (31751003), the Health Commission of Zhejiang Province (2022KY168) and the Beijing Bethune Charitable Foundation (BJ-GY2021013J).

Institutional Review Board Statement: The study was conducted in accordance with the Declaration of Helsinki and was approved by the Ethics Committee of Second Affiliated Hospital, Zhejiang University School of Medicine.

Informed Consent Statement: Patient consent was waived due to the fact that this study is retrospective.

Data Availability Statement: Not applicable.

Conflicts of Interest: The authors declare no conflict of interest.

References

1. Blankenship, G.W.; Machemer, R. Long-term diabetic vitrectomy results: Report of 10 year follow-up. *Ophthalmology* **1985**, *92*, 503–506. [CrossRef]
2. Potemkin, V.; Astakhov, S.; Goltsman, E.; Yuan, V.S. Limbal mini-pockets for transscleral IOL fixation. *Adv. Ophthalmol. Pract. Res.* **2022**, *2*, 100044. [CrossRef]
3. Sudan, R.; Muralidhar, R.; Sharma, V. Healon5 sandwich technique for phacoemulsification in vitrectomized eyes. *J. Cataract. Refract. Surg.* **2008**, *34*, 18–20. [CrossRef]
4. Dada, T.; Mandal, S.; Aggarwal, A.; Gadia, R. Microincision cataract surgery in a vitrectomized eye. *J. Cataract. Refract. Surg.* **2007**, *33*, 577–579. [CrossRef] [PubMed]
5. Cheung, C.M.; Hero, M. Stabilization of anterior chamber depth during phacoemulsification cataract surgery in vitrectomized eyes. *J. Cataract. Refract. Surg.* **2005**, *31*, 2055–2057. [CrossRef] [PubMed]
6. Chang, M.A.; Parides, M.K.; Chang, S.; Braunstein, R.E. Outcome of phacoemulsification after pars plana vitrectomy. *Ophthalmology* **2002**, *109*, 948–954. [CrossRef]
7. Ahfat, F.G.; Yuen, C.H.W.; Groenewald, C.P. Phacoemulsification and intraocular lens implantation following pars plana vitrectomy: A prospective study. *Eye* **2003**, *17*, 16–20. [CrossRef] [PubMed]
8. Tajunisah, I.; Reddy, S.C. Dropped nucleus following phacoemulsification cataract surgery. *Med. J. Malaysia* **2007**, *62*, 364–367.
9. Zauberman, H. Extreme Deepening of the Anterior Chamber During Phacoemulsification. *Ophthalmic Surg. Lasers Imaging Retin.* **1992**, *23*, 555–556. [CrossRef]
10. Wilbrandt, H.R.; Wilbrandt, T.H. Pathogenesis and management of the lens-iris diaphragm retropulsion syndrome during phacoemulsification. *J. Cataract. Refract. Surg.* **1994**, *20*, 48–53. [CrossRef]
11. Grusha, Y.; Masket, S.; Miller, K. Phacoemulsification and lens implantation after pars plana vitrectomy. *Ophthalmology* **1998**, *105*, 287–294. [CrossRef]
12. Ghosh, S.; Best, K.; Steel, D.H. Lens–iris diaphragm retropulsion syndrome during phacoemulsification in vitrectomized eyes. *J. Cataract. Refract. Surg.* **2013**, *39*, 1852–1858. [CrossRef] [PubMed]
13. Aaberg, T.M. Clinical Results in Vitrectomy for Diabetic Traction Retinal Detachment. *Am. J. Ophthalmol.* **1979**, *88*, 246–253. [CrossRef]
14. McDermott, M.L.; Puklin, J.E.; Abrams, G.W.; Eliott, D. Phacoemulsification for Cataract Following Pars Plana Vitrectomy. *Ophthalmic Surg. Lasers Imaging Retin.* **1997**, *28*, 558–564. [CrossRef]
15. Smiddy, W.E.; Stark, W.J.; Michels, R.G.; Maumenee, A.E.; Terry, A.C.; Glaser, B.M. Cataract Extraction after Vitrectomy. *Ophthalmology* **1987**, *94*, 483–487. [CrossRef]
16. Kang, Y.K.; Kim, M.J.; Kim, H.K.; Chun, B.Y. Clinical Analysis of Ocular Parameters Contributing to Intraoperative Pain during Standard Phacoemulsification. *J. Ophthalmol.* **2017**, *2017*, 9463871. [CrossRef]
17. Szijártó, Z.; Haszonits, B.; Biró, Z.; Kovács, B. Phacoemulsification on Previously Vitrectomized Eyes: Results of a 10-Year Period. *Eur. J. Ophthalmol.* **2007**, *17*, 601–604. [CrossRef]
18. Hocaoglu, M.; Karacorlu, M.; Sayman Muslubas, I.; Ozdemir, H.; Arf, S.; Uysal, O. Incidence and factors associated with com-plications of sutured and sutureless cataract surgery following pars plana vitrectomy at a tertiary referral centre in Turkey. *Br. J. Ophthalmol.* **2016**, *100*, 1206–1210. [CrossRef] [PubMed]
19. Pardo-Muñoz, A.; Muriel-Herrero, A.; Abraira, V.; Muriel, A.; Muñoz-Negrete, F.; Murube, J. Phacoemulsification in Previously Vitrectomized Patients: An Analysis of the Surgical Results in 100 Eyes as well as the Factors Contributing to the Cataract Formation. *Eur. J. Ophthalmol.* **2006**, *16*, 52–59. [CrossRef]

20. Sachdev, N.; Brar, G.S.; Sukhija, J.; Gupta, V.; Ram, J. Phacoemulsification in vitrectomized eyes: Results using a 'phaco chop' technique. *Acta Ophthalmol.* **2009**, *87*, 382–385. [CrossRef] [PubMed]
21. Misra, A.; Burton, R.L. Incidence of intraoperative complications during phacoemulsification in vitrectomized and nonvitrectomized eyes: Prospective study. *J. Cataract. Refract. Surg.* **2005**, *31*, 1011–1014. [CrossRef] [PubMed]
22. Treumer, F.; Bunse, A.; Rudolf, M.; Roider, J. Pars plana vitrectomy, phacoemulsification and intraocular lens implantation. Comparison of clinical complications in a combined versus two-step surgical approach. *Graefe's Arch. Clin. Exp. Ophthalmol.* **2005**, *244*, 808–815. [CrossRef] [PubMed]
23. Lee, J.Y.; Kim, K.-H.; Shin, K.H.; Han, D.H.; Lee, D.Y.; Nam, D.H. Comparison of Intraoperative Complications of Phacoemulsification between Sequential and Combined Procedures of Pars Plana Vitrectomy and Cataract Surgery. *Retina* **2012**, *32*, 2026–2033. [CrossRef]
24. Cole, C.J.; Charteris, D.G. Cataract extraction after retinal detachment repair by vitrectomy: Visual outcome and complications. *Eye* **2009**, *23*, 1377–1381. [CrossRef]
25. Valesova, L.; Hyel, J.; Diblik, P. [Phacoemulsification of cataracts after pars plana vitrectomy (comparison of phacoemulsifi-cation with pars plana infusion and without pars plana infusion)]. *Cesk. Slov. Oftalmol.* **2004**, *60*, 139–142. [PubMed]
26. Blumenthal, M.; Assia, E.I.; Chen, V.; Avni, I. Using an anterior chamber maintainer to control intraocular pressure during phacoemulsification. *J. Cataract. Refract. Surg.* **1994**, *20*, 93–96. [CrossRef]
27. Wahab, S.; Faiz-ur-Rab, K.; Hargun, L.D. Outcome of dual infusion through irrigating chopper in conventional phacoemulsification. *J. Pak. Med. Assoc.* **2011**, *61*, 145–148. [PubMed]
28. Hoffman, R.S.; Fine, I.H.; Packer, M. New phacoemulsification technology. *Curr. Opin. Ophthalmol.* **2005**, *16*, 38–43. [CrossRef] [PubMed]
29. Joshi, R.S. Phaco-emulsification in completely vitrectomized eyes: Intraoperative analysis of modified phaco sleeve. *Indian J. Ophthalmol.* **2016**, *64*, 659–662. [CrossRef] [PubMed]

Journal of
Personalized
Medicine

MDPI

Article

Could Mid- to Late-Onset Glaucoma Be Associated with an Increased Risk of Incident Dementia? A Nationwide Retrospective Cohort Study

Dong-Kyu Kim [1,2,*] and So Yeon Lee [3]

1 Institute of New Frontier Research, Division of Big Data and Artificial Intelligence, Chuncheon Sacred Heart Hospital, Hallym University College of Medicine, Chuncheon 24252, Republic of Korea
2 Department of Otorhinolaryngology-Head and Neck Surgery, Chuncheon Sacred Heart Hospital, Hallym University College of Medicine, Chuncheon 24252, Republic of Korea
3 Department of Ophthalmology, Nune Eye Hospital, Seoul 06198, Republic of Korea
* Correspondence: doctordk@naver.com; Tel.: +82-33-240-5180

Abstract: This study aimed to investigate the possible link between glaucoma and dementia using a nationwide cohort sample of data. The glaucoma group (n = 875) included patients diagnosed between 2003 and 2005, aged over 55 years; the comparison group was selected using propensity score matching (n = 3500). The incidence of all-cause dementia was 18.67 (7014.7 person-years) among those with glaucoma aged over 55 years. The glaucoma group developed all-cause dementia more frequently than those in the comparison group (adjusted hazard ratio (HR) = 1.43, 95% confidence interval (CI), 1.17–1.74). In a subgroup analysis, primary open-angle glaucoma (POAG) showed a significantly increased adjusted HR for all-cause dementia events (1.52, 95% CI: 1.23–1.89), whereas we could not find any significant association in patients with primary angle-closure glaucoma (PACG). Additionally, POAG patients showed an increased risk of the development of Alzheimer's disease (adjusted HR = 1.57, 95% CI, 1.21–2.04) and Parkinson's disease (adjusted HR = 2.29, 95% CI, 1.46–3.61), but there was no significant difference in PACG patients. Moreover, the risk of Alzheimer's disease and Parkinson's disease was higher within 2 years of POAG diagnosis. Although our findings have some limitations, such as confounding factor bias, we suggest that clinicians should pay attention to the early detection of dementia in patients with POAG.

Keywords: glaucoma; dementia; Alzheimer's; Parkinson's; risk

Citation: Kim, D.-K.; Lee, S.Y. Could Mid- to Late-Onset Glaucoma Be Associated with an Increased Risk of Incident Dementia? A Nationwide Retrospective Cohort Study. *J. Pers. Med.* **2023**, *13*, 214. https://doi.org/10.3390/jpm13020214

Academic Editors: Kai Jin and Chun Zhang

Received: 29 December 2022
Revised: 24 January 2023
Accepted: 25 January 2023
Published: 26 January 2023

1. Introduction

Glaucoma is characterized by optic neuropathy with progressive degeneration of retinal ganglion cells, which represents the visual field defect [1]. Its typical symptoms are a gradual loss of peripheral vision that is followed by progressive loss of central vision. Although early detection and management of glaucoma can alleviate the disease status and economic burdens of glaucoma greatly, early-stage glaucoma generally is asymptomatic; thus, it is a major leading cause of blindness in the developed world [2]. It mostly affects adults over 40, but young adults, children, and even infants can have it. Currently, the two most common forms of glaucoma are primary open-angle glaucoma (POAG) and primary angle-closure glaucoma (PACG). The goal of glaucoma treatment is to maintain the patient's visual function and related quality of life at a sustainable cost. Thus, the cost of treatment in terms of inconvenience and side effects, as well as financial implications for the individual and society, requires careful evaluation. On these days, most patients with early to moderate glaucoma damage could have suitable visual function and a modest reduction in quality of life. Dementia is a neurodegenerative disease group in which there is deterioration in cognitive function beyond what might be expected from the usual consequences of biological aging. Among those, Alzheimer's disease and Parkinson's disease are the most common type of dementia [3], whereas these usually show a long asymptomatic period. Thus, at the time of diagnosis, affected patients often suffered from extensive and irreversible damage [4]. Like other progressive brain diseases, they are associated with a buildup of certain proteins in the brain. Generally, Alzheimer's disease always causes dementia, whereas Parkinson's disease, a movement disorder, can sometimes cause dementia. For these reasons, both glaucoma and dementia have common pathologic features in terms of neurodegenerative conditions characterized by neuronal loss leading to cognitive and visual dysfunction, respectively. Additionally, both diseases become more prevalent according to increased age. To date, due to certain pathogenic and age-prevalence similarities, several epidemiologic studies have shown the potential risk of developing dementia in patients with glaucoma [5–7]. One Taiwan cohort study reported that POAG is a significant predictor for the development of Alzheimer's disease, but POAG is not a predictor of Parkinson's disease [5]. Other Taiwan cohort studies also described that female dementia patients showed a higher proportion of prior POAG than controls [6]. Meanwhile, one cohort study from South Korea revealed that POAG was associated with an increased risk of developing Alzheimer's disease; however, there was no positive association between POAG and Parkinson's disease [7]. However, these studies have some critical limitations regarding study design, including the presence of wash-our period, diagnosis age of glaucoma, and the date of enrolment. Therefore, to further investigate the relationship between the two diseases, we examined the association of mid- to late-onset glaucoma with the prospective risk of dementia using a representative sample from the National Sample Cohort data in the Republic of Korea.

2. Materials and Methods

This study was also approved by the Institutional Review Board of Hallym Medical University Chuncheon Sacred Hospital (IRB No. 2022-09-001), and the need for written informed consent was waived because the Korean National Health Insurance Service cohort (KNHIS) data set consisted of deidentified secondary data for research purposes. In terms of data availability, the authors confirm that the data supporting the findings of this study are available within the article.

2.1. Database

South Korea has had a single-payer national health system covering the entire Republic of the Korean population since 1989. An insured individual pays for national health insurance, which is proportional to the individual's income, and each Republic of Korea is assigned a unique identification number at birth. With the integration of medical aid data into the KNHIS database in 2006, this database comprises the entire population of the Republic of Korea. For these reasons, the claims data in the KNHIS cannot be omitted or duplicated. Therefore, usage of the KNHIS database eliminates selection bias. Additionally, all disease diagnostic codes were identified using the Korean Classification of Disease, Fifth Edition modification of the International Classification of Disease and Related Health Problems, 10th revision (ICD-10). Thus, in this study, we utilized a database of the representative cohort sample consisting of 1,025,340 adults obtained from the KNHIS healthcare claims data. In 2002, we conducted stratified random sampling was performed among the Republic of Korea population of 46 million with 1476 strata by age (18 groups), sex (two groups), and income levels (41 groups: 40 health insurance and one medical aid beneficiary). Thus, we investigated the present study using the KNHIS database collected from 2002 to 2013, comprising information from a nationally representative sample of 1,025,340 random individuals, accounting for approximately 2.2% of the Republic of the Korean population in 2002.

2.2. Study Design

Briefly, Figure 1 shows the study design and the process of enrolment for the study participants. We had a washout period of one year (January to December 2002) to exclude those with a risk of developing dementia before glaucoma diagnosis. First, the glaucoma group was defined as the presence of diagnostic code (H40.1 and H40.2) more than two times within the index period and over age 55 years. These cases of POAG were all diagnosed by certified ophthalmologists. We also excluded patients (1) aged < 55 years, (2) who died during the index period, and (3) diagnosed with dementia before glaucoma diagnosis. Next, we identified non-glaucoma participants as a comparison group (non-glaucoma) using propensity score-matching methodology from the remaining cohort registered in the database as four participants without cancer for each cancer patient. Additionally, we selected each participant in the comparison group who matched with each patient in the glaucoma group in terms of all independent variables and the date of enrolment (glaucoma diagnosis). The primary endpoints in this study were defined as the specific event (dementia: Alzheimer's [F00, G30], Parkinson's disease [G20], other types of dementia [F01, F02, F03]) until 31 December 2013. If patients had no events until the final following period of this database, we censored this time point. In this study, to elaborate the analysis, we set some patients' detailed characteristics as dependent variables (age, sex, residence, and household income). Additionally, we obtained information on the comorbidities of each individual and categorized the comorbidities using the Charlson comorbidity index (CCI), which is a weighted index of categorizing comorbidities of patients. The CCI is a weighted index to predict the risk of death within 1 year of hospitalization for patients with specific comorbid conditions. Nineteen conditions were included in the index. All independent variables are classified as follows: age (55–64, ≥65 years), sex (male, female), residence (Seoul, the largest metropolitan region in South Korea; 2nd area: other metropolitan cities in the Republic of Korea; and 3rd area: small cities and rural areas), household income (low: ≤30%, middle: 30.1–69.9%, and high: ≥70% of the median), and three comorbidity status (CCI: 0, 1, ≥2).

2.3. Statistical Analysis

We assessed the incidence rate as a measure of the frequency with which a specific disease or other incident events appears over a certain period. The overall incidence was expressed as per 1000 person-years, which is the following three cases: First, if the participant died, the number of years from the initial specific events diagnosis to the date of death; second, if specific events appeared, the number of years from the initial glaucoma diagnosis to the date of the first diagnosis of specific events; finally, if there are no events, the number of years from the date of initial cancer diagnosis to the final following period. Additionally, we used Cox proportional hazard regression analyses to calculate the hazard ratio (HR) and 95% confidence intervals (CI), adjusted for the other independent variables. During the follow-up period, the Kaplan–Meier method was used to calculate the specific disease-free survival rates among groups. All statistical analyses were performed using R version 4.0.5 (URL https://www.R-project.org/ accessed on 1 March 2021). p-values of <0.05 were considered statistically significant.

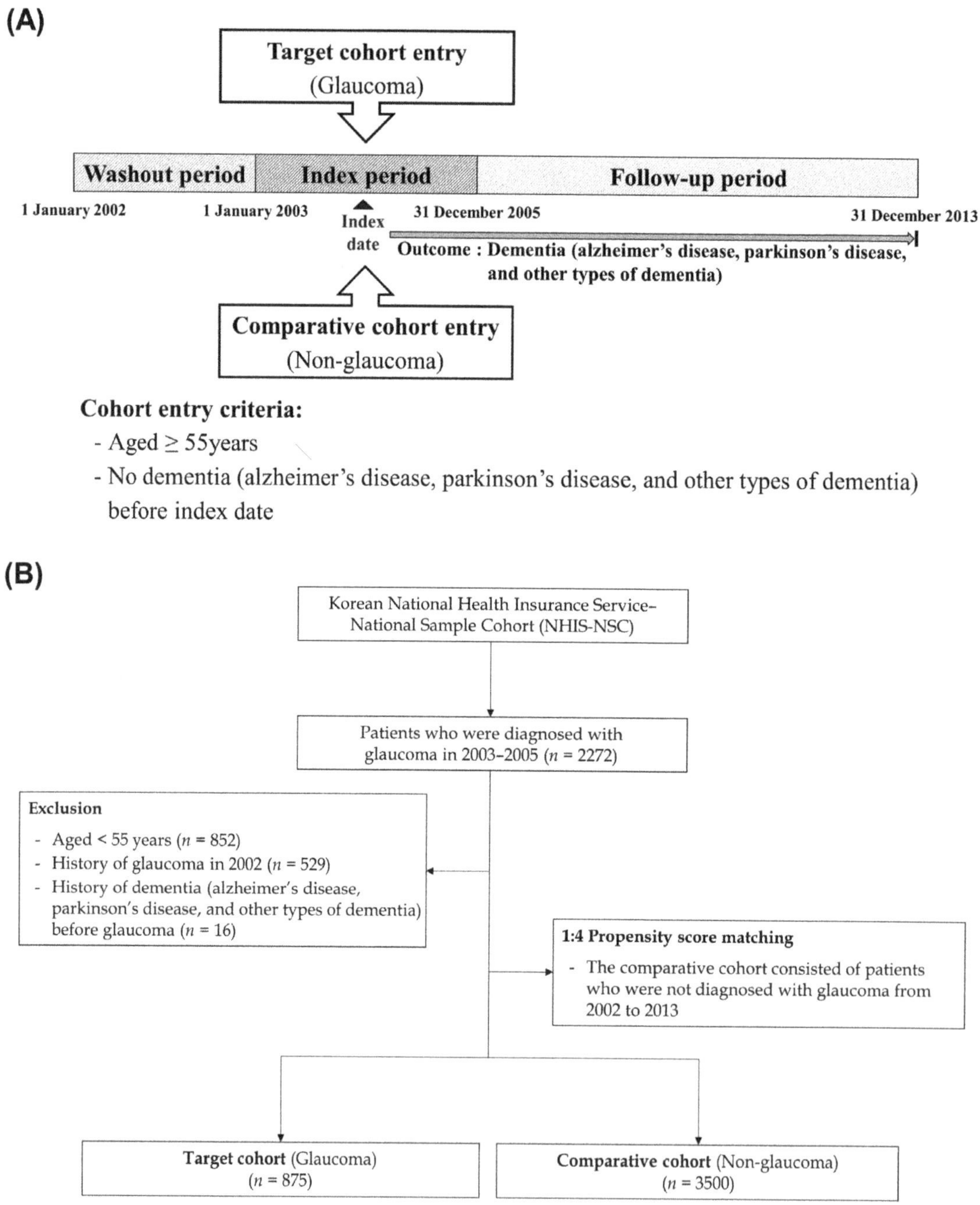

Figure 1. (**A**) Schematic study design; (**B**) process of study enrolment.

3. Results

The present study consisted of 875 participants with mid- to late-onset glaucoma and 3500 participants without glaucoma. We followed these participants in both groups for 10 years. We also confirmed that the distributions of all independent variables were similar between the groups using the balance plot technique. It indicated that the matching between the two groups was appropriate. The detailed characteristics of the study participants in each group are shown in Table 1.

Table 1. Characteristics of the study participants in each group.

Variables	Comparison (n = 3500)	Glaucoma (n = 875)	p-Value
Sex			1.000
Male	1572 (44.9%)	393 (44.9%)	
Female	1928 (55.1%)	482 (55.1%)	
Ages (years)			1.000
55–64	1424 (40.7%)	356 (40.7%)	
≥65	2076 (59.3%)	519 (59.3%)	
Residence			1.000
Seoul	724 (20.7%)	181 (20.7%)	
Second area	820 (23.4%)	205 (23.4%)	
Third area	1956 (55.9%)	489 (55.9%)	
Household income			1.000
Low (0–30%)	704 (20.1%)	176 (20.1%)	
Middle (30–70%)	1172 (33.5%)	293 (33.5%)	
High (70–100%)	1624 (46.4%)	406 (46.4%)	
CCI			1.000
0	1660 (47.4%)	415 (47.4%)	
1	900 (25.7%)	225 (25.7%)	
≥2	940 (26.9%)	235 (26.9%)	

In this study, 7014.7 person-years in the glaucoma group and 2893.5 person-years in the comparison group were evaluated for dementia events. The overall incidence of dementia was evaluated at 18.67 per 1000 person-years in the glaucoma group (Table 2). Additionally, for subgroup analysis, we assessed Alzheimer's disease, Parkinson's disease, and other types of dementia. We detected that, in the glaucoma group, the overall incidence was 11.85 in Alzheimer's disease, 4.25 in Parkinson's disease, and 7.88 in other types of dementia, respectively (Table 2). All subgroups showed a higher incidence rate of each subtype of dementia in mid- to late-onset glaucoma patients than in comparison.

Table 2. The incidence rate of dementia between glaucoma and comparison (non glaucoma) groups.

Variables	N	Case	Person Year	Incidence
		Dementia		
Comparison	3500	393	28,935.3	13.58
Glaucoma	875	131	7014.7	18.67
		Alzheimer's disease		
Comparison	3500	251	29,411.2	8.53
Glaucoma	875	85	7175.5	11.85
		Parkinson's disease		
Comparison	3500	61	29,776.4	2.05
Glaucoma	875	31	7294.7	4.25
		Other types of dementia		
Comparison	3500	194	29,504.8	6.58
Glaucoma	875	57	7231.1	7.88

We analyzed the risk of the subsequent development of dementia using univariate and multivariate Cox regression models (Table 3). After adjusting for all independent variables, we found that glaucoma was significantly associated with the development of dementia (adjusted HR = 1.43, 95% CI, 1.17–1.74). The risk of incident dementia events is also significantly increased in POAG patients but not in PACG patients.

Table 3. The risk of incident dementia events between mid- to late-life glaucoma and comparison (non-glaucoma) groups.

Variables	N	Case	Unadjusted HR (95% CI)	Adjusted HR (95% CI)
Comparison	3500	393	1.00 (ref)	1.00 (ref)
Glaucoma	875	131	1.44 (1.18–1.75) ***	1.43 (1.17–1.74) ***
POAG	695	109	1.52 (1.23–1.88) ***	1.52 (1.23–1.89) ***
PACG	180	22	1.13 (0.74–1.74)	1.08 (0.70–1.66)

POAG, primary open-angle glaucoma; PACG, primary angle-closure glaucoma; HR, hazard ratio; CI, confidence interval. *** $p < 0.001$.

In Figure 3, we detected that patients with POAG showed a significantly increased risk for dementia development, but there was no association in PACG patients. Additionally, when we investigated the risk of dementia according to subtype, we found that POAG patients were significantly associated with the development of Alzheimer's disease (adjusted HR = 1.57, 95% CI, 1.21–2.04) and Parkinson's disease (adjusted HR = 2.29, 95% CI, 1.46–3.61); however, there was no significant difference in the risk of each subtype of dementia in PACG patients (Figure 2). Meanwhile, other types of dementia showed no association in both POAG or PACG patients.

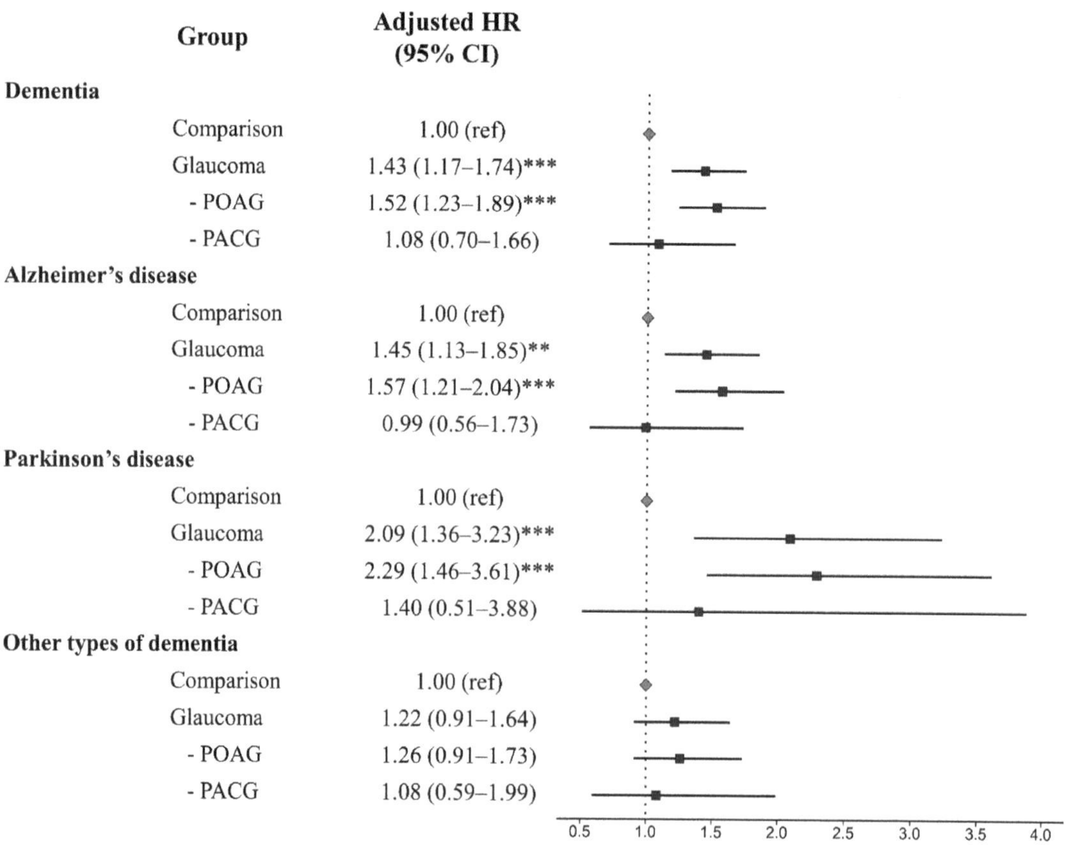

Figure 2. The adjusted hazard ratio plot of each dementia subtype among groups. POAG, primary open-angle glaucoma; PACG, primary angle-closure glaucoma; HR, hazard ratio; CI, confidence interval. ** $p < 0.010$ and *** $p < 0.001$.

The Kaplan–Meier survival analysis revealed that patients in the glaucoma group, specifically in POAG, presented a more frequent incidence of all-cause dementia, Alzheimer's disease, and Parkinson's disease events than those in the control group (Figure 3).

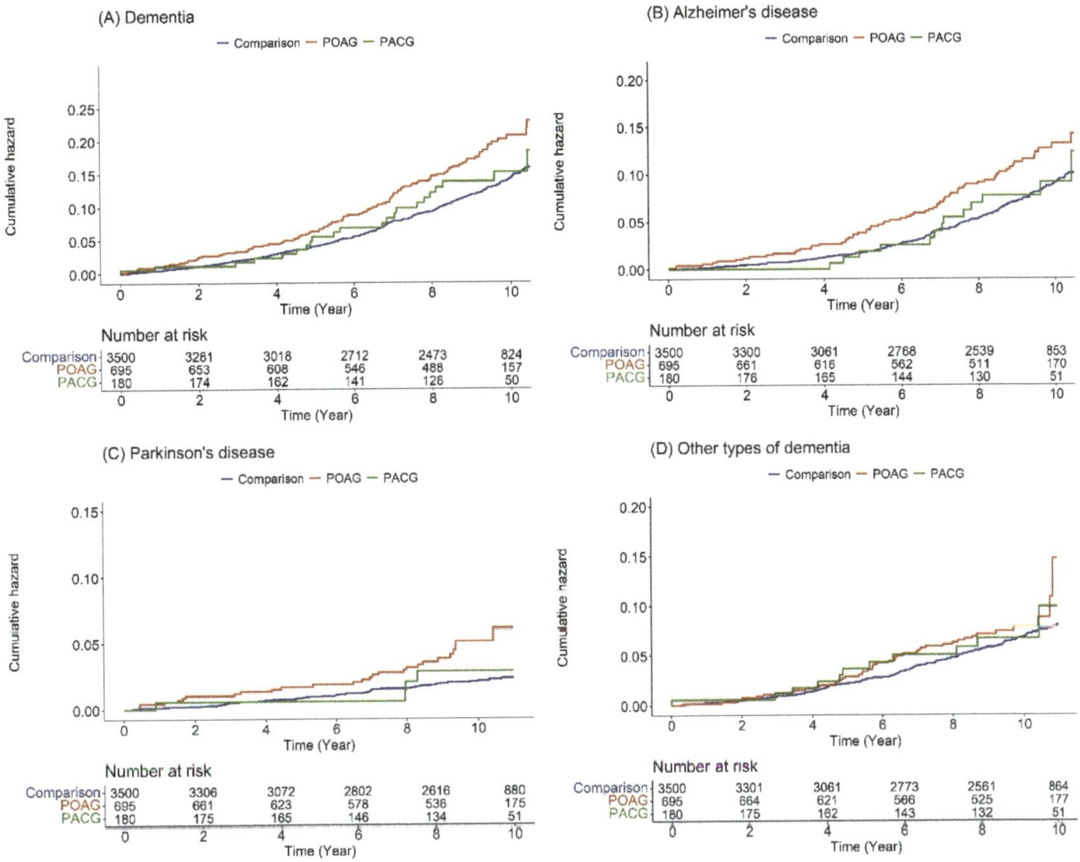

Figure 3. Cumulative hazard plot of specific diseases among comparison, POAG, and PACG: (**A**) dementia; (**B**) Alzheimer's disease; (**C**) Parkinson's disease; (**D**) other types of dementia. POAG, primary open-angle glaucoma; PACG, primary angle-closure glaucoma.

Moreover, in the analysis of HRs over time, the risk of Alzheimer's disease and Parkinson's disease development in patients with POAG was higher within two years after glaucoma diagnosis (Table 4). Meanwhile, two years after glaucoma diagnosis, the risk level of Alzheimer's disease and Parkinson's disease development in POAG patients showed similar during the follow-up period.

Table 4. Risk of dementia subtype in primary open-angle glaucoma (POAG) patients by time.

Time (Year)	Dementia		Alzheimer's Disease		Parkinson's Disease		Other Types of Dementia	
	No. of Event	Adjusted HR (95% CI)	No. of Event	Adjusted HR (95% CI)	No. of Event	Adjusted HR (95% CI)	No. of Event	Adjusted HR (95% CI)
1	7	2.03 (0.84–4.90)	4	4.07 (1.09–15.19) *	3	2.88 (0.69–12.07)	1	0.64 (0.08–5.11)
2	16	2.16 (1.20–3.89) *	8	2.69 (1.14–6.36) *	7	4.29 (1.55–11.84) **	4	1.26 (0.42–3.76)
3	22	1.69 (1.04–2.75) *	11	2.25 (1.10–4.57) *	7	1.99 (0.83–4.81)	8	1.36 (0.62–2.99)
4	29	1.55 (1.02–2.36) *	17	2.20 (1.25–3.90) **	9	2.01 (0.92–4.37)	11	1.22 (0.63–2.37)
5	40	1.58 (1.11–2.25) *	24	2.19 (1.36–3.55) **	11	2.03 (1.00–4.09) *	18	1.31 (0.78–2.20)
6	54	1.63 (1.20–2.21) **	33	2.05 (1.37–3.08) ***	12	1.73 (0.90–3.35)	26	1.52 (0.98–2.36)
7	68	1.50 (1.14–1.97) **	41	1.70 (1.19–2.42) **	15	1.74 (0.96–3.14)	32	1.36 (0.92–2.01)
8	84	1.59 (1.24–2.03) ***	53	1.74 (1.27–2.38) ***	19	2.00 (1.17–3.42) *	37	1.33 (0.92–1.91)
9	94	1.48 (1.18–1.86) ***	62	1.60 (1.20–2.12) **	22	1.95 (1.19–3.20) **	41	1.25 (0.89–1.76)
10	103	1.49 (1.19–1.85) ***	67	1.52 (1.16–2.00) **	26	2.25 (1.42–3.57) ***	43	1.20 (0.86–1.68)
11	109	1.52 (1.23–1.89) ***	72	1.57 (1.21–2.04) ***	27	2.29 (1.46–3.61) ***	46	1.26 (0.91–1.73)

HR, hazard ratio; CI, confidence interval. * $p < 0.05$, ** $p < 0.010$, and *** $p < 0.001$.

Table 5. Risk of Alzheimer's disease and Parkinson's disease in POAG patients according to the sex.

Sex	Male		Female	
	Comparison	POAG	Comparison	POAG
		Alzheimer's disease		
Unadjusted HR (95% CI)	1.00 (ref)	1.31 (0.92–1.85)	1.00 (ref)	2.18 (1.45–3.27) ***
Adjusted HR (95% CI)	1.00 (ref)	1.27 (0.90–1.81)	1.00 (ref)	2.16 (1.43–3.24) ***
		Parkinson's disease		
Unadjusted HR (95% CI)	1.00 (ref)	3.01 (1.70–5.36) ***	1.00 (ref)	1.57 (0.74–3.33)
Adjusted HR (95% CI)	1.00 (ref)	2.94 (1.65–5.23) ***	1.00 (ref)	1.57 (0.74–3.33)

*** $p < 0.001$.

Furthermore, we performed the subgroup analysis of HRs according to sex and comorbidities. We detected that the risk of Alzheimer's disease was higher in female patients with POAG, whereas male patients showed a higher risk of Parkinson's disease (Table 5). In terms of comorbidities, the adjusted HR of Alzheimer's disease and Parkinson's disease development in POAG patients was significantly increased in the comorbidities group compared to the non-comorbidities group (Table 6).

Table 6. Risk of Alzheimer's disease and Parkinson's disease in POAG patients according to the comorbidities.

CCI	0		1		≥2	
	Comparison	**POAG**	**Comparison**	**POAG**	**Comparison**	**POAG**
			Alzheimer's disease			
Unadjusted HR (95% CI)	1.00 (ref)	1.51 (0.88–2.60)	1.00 (ref)	1.87 (1.12–3.10) *	1.00 (ref)	1.49 (1.03–2.17) *
Adjusted HR (95% CI)	1.00 (ref)	1.52 (0.88–2.61)	1.00 (ref)	1.84 (1.11–3.05) *	1.00 (ref)	1.47 (1.01–2.14) *
			Parkinson's disease			
Unadjusted HR (95% CI)	1.00 (ref)	1.43 (0.57–3.57)	1.00 (ref)	1.78 (0.70–4.48)	1.00 (ref)	3.52 (1.84–6.77) ***
Adjusted HR (95% CI)	1.00 (ref)	1.41 (0.57–3.53)	1.00 (ref)	1.75 (0.69–4.43)	1.00 (ref)	3.48 (1.81–6.69) ***

POAG, primary open-angle glaucoma; CCI, Charlson comorbidity index; HR, hazard ratio; CI, confidence interval. * $p < 0.05$ and *** $p < 0.001$.

4. Discussion

Evidence obtained from many previous studies may show a possible link between two diseases based on potential pathophysiological mechanisms. To our knowledge, the epidemiologic relationship between neurodegenerative diseases and glaucoma has been widely investigated. Although some studies have not found an increased risk of dementia in patients with glaucoma [8,9], many studies have demonstrated that POAG has a potentially increased risk of Alzheimer's disease [5–7]. However, some limitations of these epidemiologic studies were that there was no washout period to eliminate the preexisting dementias, glaucoma patients include a relatively young age, and the matching control group is not clear. In this study, using longitudinal data from a nationwide cohort, we demonstrated an increased risk of not only Alzheimer's disease but also Parkinson's disease development in POAG patients aged over 55 years during a 10-year follow-up period compared with a comparison group (non-glaucoma). Interestingly, we also found that patients with POAG showed a higher risk of Alzheimer's disease and Parkinson's disease development within two years after glaucoma diagnosis. Two years later, on glaucoma diagnosis, the risk level of Alzheimer's disease and Parkinson's disease development in POAG patients slightly decreased and then continued to a constant level during the follow-up period.

It is known that various evidence exists possible linking between the two diseases, including structural abnormalities, specifically degenerative changes within ganglion cells. Besides Similar degenerative changes, neurodegenerative diseases and POAG have possible overlapping pathophysiologic mechanisms. Although the exact pathogenesis is still unclear, elevated intraocular pressure (IOP) is a major risk factor for the development and progression of POAG [10]. The difference in IOP and CSF pressure across the lamina cribrosa, the translaminar pressure difference, is an important factor in causing more optic nerve damage [11,12]. Additionally, some neurotoxic substances such as β-amyloid and tau protein were observed in both neurodegenerative disease and glaucoma [13–15]. Another possible explanation for the possible link between the two diseases is that vascular factors, such as hypertension, DM, and hyperlipidemia, are one of the major risk factors for developing each disease [16–18]. Similar to previous reports, [5–7] our findings showed the association between POAG and Alzheimer's disease. However, contrary to these reports, we also find the increased subsequent development of Parkinson's disease in POAG.

Parkinson's disease is most commonly known for affecting function and movement, though it also affects cognition, particularly as the disease progresses. It is a neurodegenerative disorder of the brain, such as Alzheimer's disease, and also has similar neurotoxic substances and vascular risk factors [19–21]. However, prior studies showed no association between POAG and Parkinson's disease during the follow-up period [5,22]. However, one study included a young age group in POAG patients, and the other study only included patients who had received anti-glaucoma medication or undergone glaucoma surgery during the study period. We thought that these issues might play a confounding variable in evaluating the risk of incident Parkinson's disease events. Thus, in the present study, we identified the risk of dementia in all glaucoma patients over 55 years who were diagnosed by certified ophthalmologists. Consistent with our findings, some studies demonstrated that Parkinson's disease was more likely to develop glaucoma-like VF defects and observed reduced RNFL thickness [23–26].

PACG is a different kind of glaucoma compared with POAG. It is known that the primary pathological cause of PACG is angle closure, and high IOP is secondarily induced due to angle closure. Thus, PACG patients commonly detected a shallow anterior chamber, thickened lens, and hyperopic refractive error. Meanwhile, the cause of POAG is mainly obstruction of the aqueous humor pathway due to trabecular meshwork degeneration. This angle closure results in the prevention of aqueous humor exit and is followed by IOP, which is thought to damage the optic nerve. PACG shows its distinctive anatomical characteristic, such as a narrow anterior chamber angle, which induces its unique pathological process [27,28]. Meanwhile, several previous cohort studies showed more association of dementia in POAG, not in PACG [5–7]. Our findings were also consistent with previous cohort studies.

Interestingly, we found that the risk of Alzheimer's disease and Parkinson's disease development was relatively higher within two years after the diagnosis of POAG. Although we could not know why the risk is higher in the early period after glaucoma diagnosis, it means that early detection of Alzheimer's disease and Parkinson's disease is clinically important to patients with POAG aged over 55 years. We also found that the risk of Alzheimer's disease and Parkinson's disease was different according to sex or comorbidities. Generally, female is nearly twice as likely as male to develop Alzheimer's disease, and the risk of developing Parkinson's disease is twice as high in males than in females. Meanwhile, it is known that comorbidity in neurodevelopmental disorders is pronounced. However, in this study, we could not determine whether these findings are a clue to a possible link between the two diseases or only a temporal incidental finding. Thus, we need further studies to prove these findings.

This study has several limitations. First, this study could not present the direct mechanism between dementia and POAG due to our study design, in which the baseline characteristics of the individuals are limited to a previous database. Thus, we could not confirm whether our findings are a causal relationship or temporal incidence. Second, the diagnosis of glaucoma and dementia was based on the ICD-10 diagnostic code, not medical records that include details such as the patient's medical history and the results of neurocognitive questionnaires. It means that we could not determine the severity of these diseases and also have a misclassification bias. At present, to overcome this issue, we only included glaucoma or dementia patients who were diagnosed by ophthalmologists or neurologists. Third, we did not consider whether patients received anti-glaucoma medication or underwent glaucoma surgery during the study period; thus, these variables may influence our findings. Fourth, in this study, the exact onset time of each disease is unclear, although we considered it as the age at the first hospital visit for each disease. Finally, in this study, we adjusted several variables, which are commonly known as these variables, that could influence the primary outcome events. Thus, the dependent variables in this study are age, sex, residence, and household income. However, other dependent variables could not adjust in this study, and then, among those, some may become confounding variables. For example, we could not adjust personal health data, including the body mass index, smoking history, and alcohol consumption, because we could not access this information. Thus, these might be played as confounding factors, and our findings inevitably have their own limitations.

Nevertheless, our study also has several unique advantages. First, our database could provide us with an effective analyze all events associated with glaucoma and dementia because this cohort had a long follow-up period and represented the Republic of Korea population. Second, the reliability of the KNHIS database has been validated, which showed a similar prevalence of 20 major diseases for each of the years assessed; thus, we are able to ascertain the reliability of the KNHIS data as "fair to good" [29–31]. Third, among databases, we just selected patients who were first diagnosed with neurodegenerative diseases by neurologists and glaucoma by ophthalmologists. We thought it enhanced the accuracy of defining the study group. Finally, this study minimized the surveillance bias on the risk of dementia in POAG patients because we selected sociodermographically matched controls in the cohort database.

5. Conclusions

In the present study, we identified the association between mid- to late-onset glaucoma and the risk of dementia after adjusting for clinical and demographic factors. Our findings suggest an increased risk of all-cause dementia, Alzheimer's disease, and Parkinson's disease events in patients with POAG aged over 55 years; however, no significant association was observed in patients with PACG aged over 55 years. Additionally, the risk of Alzheimer's disease and Parkinson's disease is relatively higher within two years of POAG diagnosis. Therefore, given the potential link between the two diseases, clinicians should be aware of the potential development of dementia in patients with POAG and recommend neurologic consulting to ensure early detection of neurodegenerative diseases during the prodromal period.

Author Contributions: Conceptualization, S.Y.L. and D.-K.K.; data acquisition, S.Y.L.; data analysis/interpretation, S.Y.L. and D.-K.K.; statistical analysis, D.-K.K.; writing—original draft preparation, S.Y.L. and D.-K.K.; writing—review and editing, supervised by all authors, under the mentorship of D.-K.K.; funding acquisition, D.-K.K. All authors have read and agreed to the published version of the manuscript.

Funding: This study was supported by a grant from the Bio & Medical Technology Development Program of the National Research Foundation (NRF) funded by the Korean government (MSIT), grant number NRF-2021R1C1C1005746.

Institutional Review Board Statement: The study was conducted in accordance with the Declaration of Helsinki and approved by the Institutional Review Board of Hallym Medical University, Chuncheon Sacred Hospital (No. 2022-09-001).

Informed Consent Statement: Patient consent was waived because the Republic of Korea National Health Insurance Service–National Sample Cohort database used in the study comprised de-identified secondary data.

Data Availability Statement: The authors confirm that the data supporting the findings of this study are available within the article.

Conflicts of Interest: The authors declare no conflict of interest.

References

1. Quigley, H.A. Glaucoma. *Lancet* **2011**, *377*, 1367–1377. [CrossRef]
2. Cedrone, C.; Mancino, R.; Cerulli, A.; Cesareo, M.; Nucci, C. Epidemiology of primary glaucoma: Prevalence, incidence, and blinding effects. *Prog. Brain Res.* **2008**, *173*, 3–14. [CrossRef]
3. Jiang, T.; Sun, Q.; Chen, S. Oxidative stress: A major pathogenesis and potential therapeutic target of antioxidative agents in Parkinson's disease and Alzheimer's disease. *Prog. Neurobiol.* **2016**, *147*, 45–60. [CrossRef] [PubMed]
4. Villemagne, V.L.; Burnham, S.; Bourgeat, P.; Brown, B.; Ellis, K.A.; Salvado, O.; Szoeke, C.; Macaulay, S.L.; Martins, R.; Maruff, P.; et al. Amyloid β deposition, neurodegeneration, and cognitive decline in sporadic Alzheimer's disease: A prospective cohort study. *Lancet Neurol.* **2013**, *12*, 357–367. [CrossRef]
5. Lin, I.-C.; Wang, Y.-H.; Wang, T.-J.; Wang, I.-J.; Shen, Y.-D.; Chi, N.-F.; Chien, L.-N. Glaucoma, Alzheimer's Disease, and Parkinson's Disease: An 8-Year Population-Based Follow-Up Study. *PLoS ONE* **2014**, *9*, e108938. [CrossRef] [PubMed]
6. Chung, S.-D.; Ho, J.-D.; Chen, C.-H.; Lin, H.-C.; Tsai, M.-C.; Sheu, J.-J. Dementia is associated with open-angle glaucoma: A population-based study. *Eye* **2015**, *29*, 1340–1346. [CrossRef]

7. Moon, J.Y.; Kim, H.J.; Park, Y.H.; Park, T.K.; Park, E.-C.; Kim, C.Y.; Lee, S.H. Association between Open-Angle Glaucoma and the Risks of Alzheimer's and Parkinson's Diseases in South Korea: A 10-year Nationwide Cohort Study. *Sci. Rep.* **2018**, *8*, 1–8. [CrossRef]
8. Ou, Y.; Grossman, D.S.; Lee, P.; Sloan, F.A. Glaucoma, Alzheimer Disease and Other Dementia: A Longitudinal Analysis. *Ophthalmic Epidemiol.* **2012**, *19*, 285–292. [CrossRef] [PubMed]
9. Kessing, L.V.; Lopez, A.G.; Andersen, P.K.; Kessing, S.V. No Increased Risk of Developing Alzheimer Disease in Patients with Glaucoma. *Eur. J. Gastroenterol. Hepatol.* **2007**, *16*, 47–51. [CrossRef]
10. Boland, M.V.; Quigley, H.A. Risk Factors and Open-angle Glaucoma: Classification and Application. *Eur. J. Gastroenterol. Hepatol.* **2007**, *16*, 406–418. [CrossRef]
11. Berdahl, J.P.; Fautsch, M.P.; Stinnett, S.S.; Allingham, R.R. Intracranial Pressure in Primary Open Angle Glaucoma, Normal Tension Glaucoma, and Ocular Hypertension: A Case–Control Study. *Investig. Ophthalmol. Vis. Sci.* **2008**, *49*, 5412–5418. [CrossRef]
12. Fleischman, D.; Berdahl, J.; Stinnett, S.S.; Fautsch, M.P.; Allingham, R.R. Cerebrospinal fluid pressure trends in diseases associated with primary open-angle glaucoma. *Acta Ophthalmol.* **2015**, *93*, e234–e236. [CrossRef]
13. Yoneda, S.; Hara, H.; Hirata, A.; Fukushima, M.; Inomata, Y.; Tanihara, H. Vitreous fluid levels of β-amyloid(1–42) and tau in patients with retinal diseases. *Jpn. J. Ophthalmol.* **2005**, *49*, 106–108. [CrossRef]
14. Gupta, N.; Fong, J.; Ang, L.C.; Yücel, Y.H. Retinal tau pathology in human glaucomas. *Can. J. Ophthalmol.* **2008**, *43*, 53–60. [CrossRef]
15. Chiasseu, M.; Vargas, J.L.C.; Destroismaisons, L.; Velde, C.V.; Leclerc, N.; Di Polo, A. Tau Accumulation, Altered Phosphorylation, and Missorting Promote Neurodegeneration in Glaucoma. *J. Neurosci.* **2016**, *36*, 5785–5798. [CrossRef]
16. Aref, A.A.; Jain, S.K.A. Senile dementia and glaucoma: Evidence for a common link. *J. Ophthalmic Vis. Res.* **2015**, *10*, 178–183. [CrossRef] [PubMed]
17. Costa, V.P.; Harris, A.; Anderson, D.; Stodtmeister, R.; Cremasco, F.; Kergoat, H.; Lovasik, J.; Stalmans, I.; Zeitz, O.; Lanzl, I.; et al. Ocular perfusion pressure in glaucoma. *Acta Ophthalmol.* **2014**, *92*, e252–e266. [CrossRef] [PubMed]
18. Chow, N.; Bell, R.D.; Deane, R.; Streb, J.W.; Chen, J.; Brooks, A.; Van Nostrand, W.; Miano, J.M.; Zlokovic, B.V. Serum response factor and myocardin mediate arterial hypercontractility and cerebral blood flow dysregulation in Alzheimer's phenotype. *Proc. Natl. Acad. Sci. USA* **2007**, *104*, 823–828. [CrossRef] [PubMed]
19. Norton, S.; E Matthews, F.; E Barnes, D.; Yaffe, K.; Brayne, C. Potential for primary prevention of Alzheimer's disease: An analysis of population-based data. *Lancet Neurol.* **2014**, *13*, 788–794. [CrossRef] [PubMed]
20. Lee, I.H.; Yu, H.; Ha, S.-S.; Son, G.M.; Park, K.J.; Lee, J.J.; Kim, D.-K. Association between Late-Onset Ménière's Disease and the Risk of Incident All-Cause Dementia. *J. Pers. Med.* **2021**, *12*, 19. [CrossRef]
21. Kwon, Y.-S.; Lee, J.-J.; Lee, S.-H.; Kim, C.; Yu, H.; Sohn, J.-H.; Kim, D.-K. Risk of Dementia in Patients Who Underwent Surgery under Neuraxial Anesthesia: A Nationwide Cohort Study. *J. Pers. Med.* **2021**, *11*, 1386. [CrossRef] [PubMed]
22. Aptel, F.; Chiquet, C.; Tamisier, R.; Sapene, M.; Martin, F.; Stach, B.; Grillet, Y.; Levy, P.; Pépin, J.-L. Association between glaucoma and sleep apnea in a large French multicenter prospective cohort. *Sleep Med.* **2014**, *15*, 576–581. [CrossRef] [PubMed]
23. Bayer, A.U.; Keller, O.N.; Ferrari, F.; Maag, K.-P. Association of glaucoma with neurodegenerative diseases with apoptotic cell death: Alzheimer's disease and Parkinson's disease. *Am. J. Ophthalmol.* **2002**, *133*, 135–137. [CrossRef] [PubMed]
24. Yenice, O.; Onal, S.; Midi, I.; Ozcan, E.; Temel, A.; I-Gunal, D. Visual field analysis in patients with Parkinson's disease. *Park. Relat. Disord.* **2008**, *14*, 193–198. [CrossRef]
25. Altintas, O.; Işeri, P.; Özkan, B.; Çağlar, Y. Correlation between retinal morphological and functional findings and clinical severity in Parkinson's disease. *Doc. Ophthalmol.* **2008**, *116*, 137–146. [CrossRef]
26. Moschos, M.M.; Tagaris, G.; Markopoulos, L.; Margetis, L.; Tsapakis, S.; Kanakis, M.; Koutsandrea, C. Morphologic Changes and Functional Retinal Impairment in Patients with Parkinson Disease without Visual Loss. *Eur. J. Ophthalmol.* **2010**, *21*, 24–29. [CrossRef]
27. Lowe, R.F. Aetiology of the anatomical basis for primary angle-closure glaucoma. Biometrical comparisons between normal eyes and eyes with primary angle-closure glaucoma. *Br. J. Ophthalmol.* **1970**, *54*, 161–169. [CrossRef]
28. Sihota, R.; Ghate, D.; Mohan, S.; Gupta, V.; Pandey, R.M.; Dada, T. Study of biometric parameters in family members of primary angle closure glaucoma patients. *Eye* **2008**, *22*, 521–527. [CrossRef]
29. Lee, S.; Cha, J.; Kim, J.-Y.; Son, G.M.; Kim, D.-K. Detection of unknown ototoxic adverse drug reactions: An electronic healthcare record-based longitudinal nationwide cohort analysis. *Sci. Rep.* **2021**, *11*, 14045. [CrossRef]
30. Lee, J.; Lee, J.S.; Park, S.-H.; Shin, S.A.; Kim, K. Cohort Profile: The National Health Insurance Service–National Sample Cohort (NHIS-NSC), South Korea. *Leuk. Res.* **2016**, *46*, dyv319. [CrossRef]
31. You, S.C.; Lee, S.; Cho, S.-Y.; Park, H.; Jung, S.; Cho, J.; Yoon, D.; Park, R.W. Conversion of National Health Insurance Service-National Sample Cohort (NHIS-NSC) Database into Observational Medical Outcomes Partnership-Common Data Model (OMOP-CDM). *Stud. Health Technol. Inform.* **2017**, *245*, 467–470. [CrossRef] [PubMed]

Journal of *Personalized Medicine*

MDPI

Article

Pneumatic Retinopexy Involving the Use of Intravitreal Air Injection and Laser Photocoagulation for Rhegmatogenous Retinal Detachment in Phakic Eyes

Tiepei Zhu [1], Zhenyang Xiang [2], Qinzhu Huang [2], Gaochun Li [2], Shenchao Guo [2] and Enhui Li [2,*]

1 Eye Center, Second Affiliated Hospital of Medical College, Zhejiang University, Hangzhou 310058, China
2 Department of Ophthalmology, Taizhou Hospital of Zhejiang Province, Taizhou 318000, China
* Correspondence: lieh@enzemed.com

Abstract: The clinical efficacy of pneumatic retinopexy (PR) using intravitreal pure air injection and laser photocoagulation for rhegmatogenous retinal detachment (RRD) remains unknown. Thirty-nine consecutive patients with RRD (39 eyes) were included in this prospective case series. All patients underwent two-step PR surgery containing pure air intravitreal injection and laser photocoagulation retinopexy during hospitalization. The main outcomes were best-corrected visual acuity (BCVA) and primary anatomic success rates after PR treatment. The mean follow-up was 18.3 ± 9.7 months, ranging from 6 to 37 months. The primary anatomic success rate was 89.7% (35/39) after PR treatment. Final reattachment of the retina was achieved in 100% of cases. Macular epiretinal membrane was developed in two patients (5.7%) among successful PR cases during the follow-up. The mean logMAR BCVA value was significantly improved from 0.94 ± 0.69 before surgery to 0.39 ± 0.41 after surgery. The average central retinal thickness was significantly thinner in the RRD eyes of macula-off patients (206.8 ± 56.13 μm) when compared with the fellow eyes (234.6 ± 48.4 μm) at the last follow-up ($p = 0.005$). This study concluded that an inpatient PR procedure with pure air injection and laser photocoagulation is a safe and effective approach to treating patients with RRD, who may achieve a high single-operation success rate and good visual acuity recovery.

Keywords: retinal detachment; pneumatic retinopexy; intravitreal injection; laser photocoagulation; retinal thickness

Citation: Zhu, T.; Xiang, Z.; Huang, Q.; Li, G.; Guo, S.; Li, E. Pneumatic Retinopexy Involving the Use of Intravitreal Air Injection and Laser Photocoagulation for Rhegmatogenous Retinal Detachment in Phakic Eyes. *J. Pers. Med.* **2023**, *13*, 328. https://doi.org/10.3390/jpm13020328

Academic Editors: Kai Jin, Chun Zhang and Ana Isabel Ramírez Sebastián

Received: 16 December 2022
Revised: 31 January 2023
Accepted: 9 February 2023
Published: 14 February 2023

1. Introduction

Rhegmatogenous retinal detachment (RRD) is potentially an acute vision-threatening disease and requires surgical intervention as early as possible. Surgical approaches commonly include scleral buckling (SB), pars plana vitrectomy (PPV), pneumatic retinopexy (PR), or combinations of these treatments [1]. Although anatomic reattachment is successful in most cases, optimal management for a vast number of RRD cases remains controversial.

PR is considered the most minimally invasive treatment for repairing simple RRD. This office-based surgery has been well accepted by retinal surgeons as an alternative option for simple RRD with superior retinal breaks [2]. A recent multicenter, randomized, controlled clinical trial was performed to compare the outcomes of PR to PPV for primary RRD, the results of which suggested that PR should be considered the first-line treatment for primary RRD meeting the study criteria [3].

The successful anatomical retinal reattachment rate of single PR treatment ranged from 50% to 90% in previous studies [3–9]. The PR procedure can be performed in one step, with the application of scleral cryopexy to retinal breaks just before intravitreal gas injection, or in a two-step manner, with initial intravitreal gas injection to flatten the detached retina, followed by either laser photocoagulation or scleral cryopexy to seal the retinal break [2]. Both procedures have been applied in previous studies, depending on the surgeon's discretion [3,5]. Thus, the efficacy of PR for simple RRD may be compounded due to the different procedures used in a study.

Scleral cryopexy has been mainly applied to retinopexy in previous PR studies [3–5,10] and expansile gas such as sulfur hexafluoride (SF6) or perfluoropropane (C_3F_8) was then injected into the vitreous to ensure the internal tamponade of the retinal breaks [3–5] However, both scleral cryopexy and injection of the expansile gas may have a higher incidence of proliferative vitreoretinopathy [11,12]. Moreover, expansile gases may be unavailable in some healthcare settings. To date, the clinical outcome of PR via laser retinopexy and pure air injection for RRD is still not well characterized.

This study aims to explore the efficacy of two-step PR in which pure air intravitreal injection and laser retinopexy are used in a consecutive series of patients with RRD. It has been reported that successful retinal reattachment can be achieved after as little as 6–8 h of gas tamponade, with an appropriate head position [13]. Thus, unlike surgeons performing traditional office-based procedures, we performed the PR treatment as an inpatient procedure to (1) maintain the appropriate head position after gas injection and adjust the position in a timely manner when the retinal break was not blocked and (2) apply laser retinopexy as early as possible after the retina was attached.

2. Materials and Methods

2.1. Design and Patients

This was a prospective case series study of consecutive patients with RRD who visited the Department of Ophthalmology of Taizhou Hospital between 1 April 2019 and 31 March 2022. The inclusion criteria were as follows: had primary RRD and had not received prior treatment; presented with one break or multiple breaks separated by less than 3 clock hour positions; phakic eye; presented superior breaks located at the 8 to 4 o'clock position; presented no or minimal PVR (grade B). The exclusion criteria were as follows: retinal break size larger than one clock hour; PVR grade C or D, or retinal star folds exerted traction on the breaks; presented retinal breaks in the inferior 4 clock hour positions of the fundus; presented a giant retinal tear or dialyses; had severe or uncontrolled glaucoma; presented cloudy media such as cataracts or vitreous hemorrhage that precluded an adequate view of the peripheral retina; and had a history of prior retinal surgeries. Patients with a physical disability or mental incompetence who could not maintain the required head position were also excluded.

All the participants included in our study underwent PR surgery containing pure air intravitreal injection and laser retinopexy. The possible benefits and risks of PR treatment were explained to the patients and informed consent was obtained from all adult patients and from the parents if the patient was younger than 18 years old, in accordance with the Helsinki Declaration, before inclusion in the study. Institutional review board approval (X20180301) for this study was obtained from the Ethics Committee of Taizhou Hospital.

2.2. Surgical Technique

Careful peripheral retinal examination with scleral depression was applied to identify any pathologic features in each patient. Laser retinopexy was performed if any lattice degeneration or retinal breaks existed in the attached retina before PR treatment. The PR procedure involves an intravitreal pure air injection first, followed by laser retinopexy when the retina is attached. The air injection was performed under topical anesthesia in the operating room. For the anterior chamber paracentesis, gentle pressure was applied with a cotton-tipped applicator to facilitate more aqueous drainage. Then, 0.6–0.8 mL of filtered sterile air was injected 3.5 mm posterior to the limbus, depending on the extent of the retinal breaks and the eye size. The usual injected gas volume was 0.6 mL; however, 0.6–0.8 mL was injected if the patient had one retinal break size larger than 2 papillary diameter (PD) or multiple breaks separated by more than 1 clock hour or high myopia; a larger air bubble or a longer duration of tamponade was required in those specific patients. Then, the placement of a gas bubble over the retinal break(s) and the perfusion of the central retinal artery were confirmed with indirect ophthalmoscopy. Anterior chamber paracentesis was repeated in the situation of marked intraocular pressure elevations. All the patients were asked to maintain a proper head position continuously during hospitalization. Retinal laser photocoagulation was administered as early as 6–8 h after air injection and a supplemental laser was applied within 1–3 days during residency. The head was tilted when the residual gas bubble obstructed the laser pathway. Usually, 3–4 rows of laser spots were made around the retinal break. All the patients were followed up at 1 week, 1 month, 3 months, and 6 months post operation, then every 6 months thereafter.

2.3. Clinical Measurements

Each patient in the study underwent a complete ophthalmologic assessment, including slit-lamp examination, fundus examination with indirect ophthalmoscopy under mydriasis, and intraocular pressure measurements. Before PR surgery, clinical data—which include sex, age, lens state, the most recent refraction data before retinal detachment, best-corrected visual acuity (BCVA), days to PR treatment, the extent of the RRD area, and the number of breaks—were recorded. The main surgical outcomes were postoperative BCVA and primary PR anatomic success rates, which were defined as the ratio of successful retinal attachment after PR treatment within 6 months post operation. PR failure was defined as the need for additional intervention (scleral buckle and/or vitrectomy) for retinal detachment after initial PR treatment. In addition, macular status was confirmed by optical coherence tomography (OCT) before and after PR surgery.

2.4. Statistical Analysis

For statistical analysis of the data, we used R software for Windows (version 3.4.3; http://www.R-project.org). The Shapiro–Wilk test was applied to assess the normal distribution of the data. Comparison of data between groups was performed using one-way analysis of variance when samples were normally distributed or the Kruskal–Wallis test when parametric statistics were not possible. The potential effects of preoperative baseline characteristics on surgical outcomes were analyzed by linear mixed-effects models using the "lem4" package. p values below 0.05 were considered statistically significant.

3. Results

A total of 39 eyes of 39 patients with RRD met the inclusion criteria; these patients were enrolled in this study. The mean age of the included patients was 51.8 ± 14.5 years (range: 14–75 years). All the patients had phakic eyes and no history of intraocular surgery. The preoperative characteristics of all patients are summarized in Table 1. Twenty-one patients (21/39) were evaluated for a grade A level of proliferative vitreoretinopathy (PVR) before surgery, and the remaining cases had PVR with a grade B level. The size of retinal breaks ranged from 0.5–4 PD. Most of the breaks were typical horseshoe-shaped tears (79.4%, 31/39), and the remaining cases were identified as round-shaped holes (20.6%, 8/39). There was no significant difference in terms of age, sex, days to surgery, or number of retinal breaks between macula-on and macula-off patients. However, there was worse visual acuity and more quadrants of detached retina in the macula-off group versus the macula-on group ($p < 0.05$).

The average follow-up was 18.3 ± 9.7 months, ranging from 6 to 37 months. The primary anatomic success rate was 89.7% (35/39) after PR treatment at the last follow-up (Figure 1), and the final reattachment rate was 100% (39/39) when combined scleral buckling or PPV surgery was applied for the failed PR cases. Among the 35 patients who had successful PR cases, 34 patients (97.1%) received only a single air injection, and 1 patient needed an additional air injection because the retina was partially attached, but the air was almost completely absorbed. For postoperative complications, one patient developed a new retinal break superiorly and shallow retinal detachment two days after the initial injection. The head position was adjusted in a timely manner to close the new break with the residual air bubble, and the retina was finally attached after supplemental laser treatment. Two patients (5.7%) with successful PR cases developed macular epiretinal membranes during the follow-up. One successful PR case developed steroid-induced glaucoma at the last follow-up, which was not included for further analysis. The four failed PR cases were all macula-off type retinal detachment, and the reasons for failure were gas bubbles under the retina (one case), missed retinal break (one case), and retinal break unblocking (two cases). All of these patients underwent additional retinal repair surgeries (PPV for three patients and scleral buckling for one patient) within one week after initial PR treatment and finally had retinal attachment during the follow-up.

Table 1. Preoperative clinical characteristics of uncomplicated RRD patients.

Subject Characteristics	Total Patients	Macula-on Patients	Macula-off Patients	p †
No. of cases	39	21	18	-
Age, years	51.8 ± 14.5	52.6 ± 10.9	50.8 ± 18.2	0.715
Female, no. (%)	19 (48.7)	11 (52.4)	8 (44.4)	0.652
Right study eye, no. (%)	21 (53.8)	11 (52.4)	10 (55.6)	0.835
Spherical equivalent refractive error, diopter	−3.80 ± 3.75	−4.44 ± 4.59	−3.31 ± 3.14	0.420
Preoperative BCVA, LogMAR *	0.94 ± 0.69	0.36 ± 0.28	1.58 ± 0.36	<0.001
Days to PR surgery ¶	12.4 ± 10.0	12.6 ± 10.3	12.3 ± 9.8	0.912
No. of breaks in detached retina	1.28 ± 0.60	1.14 ± 0.48	1.44 ± 0.70	0.106
No. of quadrants of detached retina	1.4 ± 0.50	1.17 ± 0.33	1.67 ± 0.54	0.001

* Counting fingers and hand motion: visual acuity was converted to 1.6 and 1.9 LogMAR, respectively; ¶ days to PR surgery was defined as the duration from the day of symptom onset to the day of air injection; † comparisons between macula-on and -off groups; BCVA—best corrected visual acuity; PR—pneumatic retinopexy.

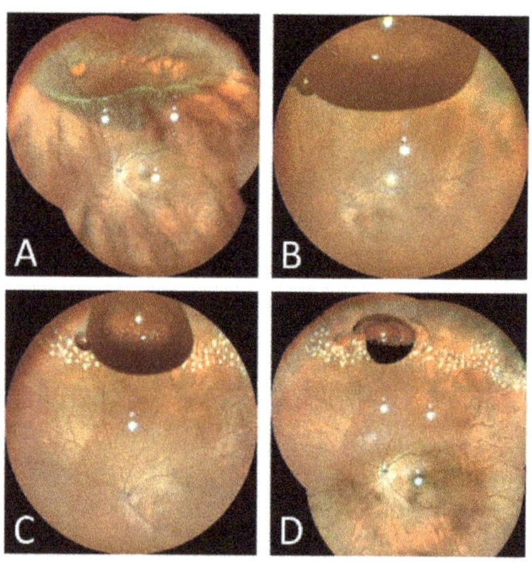

Figure 1. Fundus photography of a typical RRD case before and after PR treatment. (**A**). The patient had superior retinal detachment with multiple breaks. (**B**). The retina has completely reattached at 12 h after intravitreal air injection. (**C**) Laser retinopexy was applied the day after intravitreal air injection. (**D**) Laser retinopexy could be strengthened when the air bubble became smaller.

Postoperative best-corrected logMAR visual acuity significantly improved after retinal detachment repair surgery (Figure 2). Among successful PR cases, the preoperative BCVA of logMAR in the macula-on group was 0.37 ± 0.28 and improved to 0.16 ± 0.17 after PR treatment ($p < 0.001$, $n = 20$). The macula-off group also showed significant improvement in postoperative BCVA (1.62 ± 0.36) of logMAR over baseline (0.59 ± 0.48, $p < 0.001$, $n = 14$). The linear mixed model demonstrated that the baseline BCVA had a negative effect on the changes in BCVA, which means that the worse the baseline BCVA was, the greater the improvement achieved after surgery. In the macula-on group, no significant difference in average central retinal thickness was observed between the baseline value (236.6 ± 31.3 μm) and the postoperative eye value (231.4 ± 31.1 μm, p = 0.589, n = 16). In the macula-off group, central retinal thickness was significantly thinner in the RRD eyes (206.8 ± 56.13 μm) compared with the fellow eyes (234.6 ± 48.4 μm) at the last follow-up (p = 0.005, n = 13).

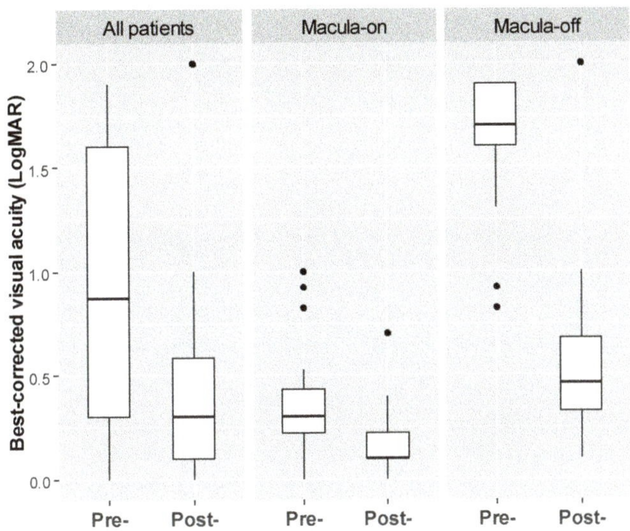

Figure 2. Box-and-whisker plot showing preoperative and postoperative best-corrected visual acuity (LogMAR) in RRD patients undergoing our two-step PR treatment.

4. Discussion

Many variations in PR treatment have been described in previous studies [2–5,7,8]. Different gas types—including C_3F_8, SF_6, and pure air can be injected, and different retinopexy approaches, such as cryopexy and laser photocoagulation, have been applied before and after gas injection. In this study, we performed a two-step PR procedure for RRD patients and further evaluated the efficacy of pure air injection followed by laser retinopexy to treat the detached retina. The outcomes demonstrated a high success rate of retinal attachment, particularly in macula-on RRD cases.

SF_6 and C_3F_8 are the gases most frequently used in the PR procedure. Because of the low solubility of these expansile gases, the average durations of SF_6 and C_3F_8 were 12 days and 38 days, respectively [10]. The prolonged longevity of expansile gas bubbles may have disadvantages. Patients need to maintain their head position for a longer period, and air travel is also prohibited. Long-lasting gas bubbles can increase the risk of cataract formation in phakic eyes [14]. Furthermore, the movement of bubbles may produce extra vitreo-retinal traction and induce new retinal breaks. Thus, nonexpansile and filtered air could be used for retinal fixation. It has been suggested that laser photocoagulation could produce mild chorioretinal adhesion within 24 h, moderate adhesion after approximately 5 to 7 days, and firm adhesion after 2 weeks [15]. A 0.8 mL intravitreal air bubble has an average duration of 4 days, which is probably sufficient time for most cases to form a moderate chorioretinal adhesion. Sinawat et al. [15] demonstrated that PR in which filtered air was used had a similar initial reattachment rate compared with that of C_3F_8 injection in a randomized noninferiority trial, although the approach of retinopexy was not mentioned in the study. Yee et al. [16] reported that office-based PR in which only pure air was used yielded a high success rate and long-term efficacy. Similarly, our study used approximately 0.6–0.8 mL of filtered air to cover the detached retina up to 120 degrees and block the retinal breaks. Unlike the expansile gas, the larger pure air bubble could reach the maximum amount immediately after initial injection and had higher buoyancy and surface tension at the early stage of PR treatment, which may facilitate epithelial pump removal of the subretinal fluid. Therefore, this initial large air bubble could allow us to treat inferior retinal detachment cases with multiple breaks separated within 2 h. Additionally, no patients had undergone RVP and one patient (1/35, 2.9%) had a new retinal break after gas injection. Two patients (2/35, 5.7%) developed macular epiretinal membranes during the follow-up, suggesting that the air injection yielded a low risk of postoperative complications.

Scleral cryopexy seems to be more commonly used in previous studies [3–5,10]. However, we performed laser retinopexy in our patients after air injection because cryopexy may be associated with a higher incidence of PVR, particularly in young patients. In addition, compared with cryopexy, lasers may produce quicker and stronger chorioretinal adhesion [17]. The use of lasers when dealing with multiple or large retinal breaks is also superior. In our inpatient PR treatment, laser photocoagulation could be performed once the retina was attached. It has been reported that successful reattachment could be achieved after as little as 6–8 h of gas injection [13], which is similar to our present results. However, if an expansile gas were used, laser application may be difficult because the gas bubble would start to expand and might impair the visualization of the retinal breaks. The single PR success rate reached 87.7% (34/39) when our procedure was used, whereas other studies reported single PR success rates of 54% and 59.4% when long-acting expansile gas was used [18,19]. In our study, the air bubbles did not expand and laser treatment was possible as early as 6 h after air injection, which was gradually finished within 3 days for our patients. Therefore, retinal breaks were blocked as soon as possible, which may be one of the reasons for the high retinal attachment rate of single PR treatment in the current study. The other reason for the high success rate may be that we performed PR treatment as an inpatient procedure, which helped us to ensure that the patients maintained the head position properly after air injection and that the position could be adjusted in a timely manner according to the status of the detached retina. In addition, postoperative complications could be noticed during hospitalization; for example, in the case of new retinal breaks after air injection, the break was treated in a timely manner, which prevented further retinal detachment.

The initial PR failed to achieve retinal attachment in four cases in our study. One of them had a missed retinal break or new break, which is suggested to be the most common cause of reoperation following PR [10]. The other failure in our series was a patient with subretinal gas following air injection, and a vitrectomy with internal drainage was performed to achieve retinal attachment. For the remaining two cases of retinal unclosed break, one patient had long axial length and very high myopia of −16 diopter; we believe the relatively unhealthy PRE pump function in the pathologic myopia patient may be the reason for persistent subretinal fluid, and vitrectomy was performed successfully to flatten the retina in this patient. In the other case, subretinal fluid shifted counterclockwise three clock hours after 8 h of head position; the fluid shift induced detachment of the inferior retina, which also had lattice degeneration before PR. The patient did not maintain proper head position at the beginning. The amount of subretinal fluid remained unchanged after 24 h of position. This failed case was further treated successfully with scleral buckle in the two days after PR surgery. Notably, because the PR affords no permanent relief of vitreoretinal traction on the break, the substantial traction after surgery may also be the reason for these two cases of PR failure.

Our study did not exclude patients without a posterior vitreous detachment. Four young patients with no posterior vitreous detachment and atrophic hole were included, and they were all successfully treated by PR in this study. Previous studies have shown the anatomic reattachment rate in pediatric RRD patients undergoing PR was similar to that reported in adult patients. Chen et al. [20] demonstrated the effectiveness of PR for retinal RRD repair in teenagers, and 84.2% of the cases were successfully reattached after one PR treatment. Additionally, Figueiredo et al. [21] found a similar reattachment rate of

85% in 20 pediatric patients undergoing PR treatment for RRD fulfilling PIVOT criteria. The younger patients may not appear to be at higher risk of failing PR. These specific cases usually have no posterior vitreous detachment and healthy RPE pump function; subretinal fluid may resolve more quickly after gas injection. Chen et al. [20] also suggested there may be less new break formation in young patients without PVD. In the condition of no PVD, the gas bubble may pose even and little traction on other parts of the retina and little chance of new break formation.

PR treatment may result in better postoperative visual acuity than other RRD repair surgeries. Tornambe et al. [22] reported that more patients achieved BCVA ≥20/40 in the PR group (81/92, 88%) versus those in the SB group (57/77, 74%). Moreover, a recent randomized controlled trial demonstrated that the visual acuity outcomes in patients undergoing PR were superior to those undergoing PPV at every follow-up timepoint. The proportion of eyes achieving ≥20/40 was 90.3% compared to 75.3% in the PPV group [3]. Yee et al. [16] showed that long-term visual outcomes following air PR showed comparable improvement with those of PR using long-lasting gases, and 87% of the patients had the same or better vision at the last follow-up. In line with previous studies, no participant had worse postoperative visual acuity in our study, and visual improvement was achieved in 76.2% (16/21) of macula-on RRD and 100% (14/14) of macula-off RRD patients.

The macular structure can be altered in RRD patients even after repair surgeries. Purtskhvanidze et al. [23] and Maqsood et al. [24] found that central retinal thickness was significantly decreased in comparison to that of controls after PPV surgery in RRD patients, especially in macula-off RRD patients. The detached retina may suffer from hypoxic conditions, the outer retinal layers may be deprived of nutrients by the subretinal fluid, and the microvasculature of the inner retinal layers may have lower blood perfusion. Nonetheless, few studies have investigated the changes in retinal structure in RRD patients after PR surgery. Kaderli et al. [25] reported that the inner retinal thickness in the eyes of macula-off RRD patients was significantly higher than that in macula-on RRD patients at 1 month and 3 months post operation. In contrast, we found significantly thinner central retinal thickness in RRD eyes than that in fellow eyes in macula-off patients. This discrepancy in results between these studies may be due to the difference in surgical techniques, follow-up time, and patient populations. We have not investigated the postoperative photoreceptor integrity on OCT images, but it has been suggested that PR treatment may be associated with less discontinuity of the ellipsoid zone and external limiting membrane at 12 months post operation, which may be the reason for the improved visual outcome after PR surgery [26].

Our study presented several limitations. The sample size was relatively small and we included only phakic eyes in the study. A future prospective randomized study with a larger number of eyes and a longer follow-up is needed to verify our findings. We have not compared our PR treatment with other RRD repair surgery treatments such as PPV or SB. A comparative prospective study comparing the outcomes of the two-step procedure of air PR with PPV and SB may yield more conclusive results.

5. Conclusions

The inpatient two-step pneumatic retinopexy with pure air injection and early laser photocoagulation may be an effective approach to treating patients with RRD, who presented a high single-operation success rate and good visual acuity recovery.

Author Contributions: Conceptualization, T.Z. and E.L.; methodology, T.Z. and E.L.; software, S.G.; formal analysis, T.Z. and S.G.; investigation, Q.H. and G.L.; resources, Z.X. and E.L.; data curation, T.Z.; writing original draft preparation, T.Z.; writing—review and editing, T.Z., Z.X., Q.H., G.L., S.G., and E.L.; visualization, T.Z.; supervision, E.L.; project administration, Z.X.; funding acquisition, T.Z. All authors have read and agreed to the published version of the manuscript.

Funding: This research was funded by the National Natural Science Foundation of China (grant number 82201197) and the Taizhou Scientific and Technological Project (grant number 1701KY53).

Institutional Review Board Statement: Institutional review board approval (X20180301) for this study was obtained from the Ethics Committee of Taizhou Hospital.

Informed Consent Statement: Informed consent was obtained from all subjects involved in the study. Written informed consent was obtained from the patients prior to the publication of this paper.

Data Availability Statement: Not applicable.

Conflicts of Interest: The authors declare no conflict of interest.

References

1. Popovic, M.M.; Muni, R.H.; Nichani, P.; Kertes, P.J. Pars plana vitrectomy, scleral buckle, and pneumatic retinopexy for the management of rhegmatogenous retinal detachment: A meta-analysis. *Surv. Ophthalmol.* **2022**, *67*, 184–196. [CrossRef] [PubMed]
2. Huang, C.Y.; Mikowski, M.; Wu, L. Pneumatic retinopexy: An update. *Graefe's Arch. Clin. Exp. Ophthalmol.* **2022**, *260*, 711–722. [CrossRef] [PubMed]
3. Hillier, R.J.; Felfeli, T.; Berger, A.R.; Wong, D.T.; Altomare, F.; Dai, D.; Giavedoni, L.R.; Kertes, P.J.; Kohly, R.P.; Muni, R.H. The Pneumatic Retinopexy versus Vitrectomy for the Management of Primary Rhegmatogenous Retinal Detachment Outcomes Randomized Trial (PIVOT). *Ophthalmology* **2019**, *126*, 531–539. [CrossRef] [PubMed]
4. Ellakwa, A.F. Long term results of pneumatic retinopexy. *Clin. Ophthalmol.* **2012**, *6*, 55–59. [CrossRef] [PubMed]
5. Fabian, I.D.; Kinori, M.; Efrati, M.; Alhalel, A.; Desatnik, H.; Hai, O.V.; Katz, G.; Platner, E.; Moisseiev, J. Pneumatic retinopexy for the repair of primary rhegmatogenous retinal detachment: A 10-year retrospective analysis. *JAMA Ophthalmol.* **2013**, *131*, 166–171. [CrossRef]
6. Vail, D.; Pan, C.; Pershing, S.; Mruthyunjaya, P. Association of rhegmatogenous retinal detachment and outcomes with the day of the week that patients undergo a repair or receive a diagnosis. *JAMA Ophthalmol.* **2020**, *138*, 156–163. [CrossRef]
7. Lee, I.T.; Lampen, S.I.R.; Wong, T.P.; Major, J.C., Jr.; Wykoff, C.C. Fovea-sparing rhegmatogenous retinal detachments: Impact of clinical factors including time to surgery on visual and anatomic outcomes. *Graefe's Arch. Clin. Exp. Ophthalmol.* **2019**, *257*, 883–889. [CrossRef]
8. Hilton, G.F.; Grizzard, W.S. Pneumatic retinopexy. A two-step outpatient operation without conjunctival incision. *Ophthalmology* **1986**, *93*, 626–641. [CrossRef]
9. Anaya, J.A.; Shah, C.P.; Heier, J.S.; Morley, M.G. Outcomes after Failed Pneumatic Retinopexy for Retinal Detachment. *Ophthalmology* **2016**, *123*, 1137–1142. [CrossRef]
10. Chan, C.K.; Lin, S.G.; Nuthi, A.S.; Salib, D.M. Pneumatic retinopexy for the repair of retinal detachments: A comprehensive review (1986–2007). *Surv. Ophthalmol.* **2008**, *53*, 443–478. [CrossRef]
11. Campochiaro, P.A.; Kaden, I.H.; Vidaurri-Leal, J.; Glaser, B.M. Cryotherapy enhances intravitreal dispersion of viable retinal pigment epithelial cells. *Arch. Ophthalmol.* **1985**, *103*, 434–436. [CrossRef]
12. Cowley, M.; Conway, B.P.; Campochiaro, P.A.; Kaiser, D.; Gaskin, H. Clinical risk factors for proliferative vitreoretinopathy. *Arch. Ophthalmol.* **1989**, *107*, 1147–1151. [CrossRef]
13. Chang, T.S.; Pelzek, C.D.; Nguyen, R.L.; Purohit, S.S.; Scott, G.R.; Hay, D. Inverted pneumatic retinopexy: A method of treating retinal detachments associated with inferior retinal breaks. *Ophthalmology* **2003**, *110*, 589–594. [CrossRef]
14. Lincoff, H.; Coleman, J.; Kreissig, I.; Richard, G.; Chang, S.; Wilcox, L.M. The perfluorocarbon gases in the treatment of retinal detachment. *Ophthalmology* **1983**, *90*, 546–551. [CrossRef]
15. Sinawat, S.; Ratanapakorn, T.; Sanguansak, T.; Prompol, S.; Laopaiboon, M.; Yospaiboon, Y. Air vs perfluoropropane gas in pneumatic retinopexy: A randomized noninferiority trial. *Arch. Ophthalmol.* **2010**, *128*, 1243–1247. [CrossRef]
16. Yee, K.M.; Sebag, J. Long-term results of office-based pneumatic retinopexy using pure air. *Br. J. Ophthalmol.* **2011**, *95*, 1728–1730. [CrossRef]
17. Folk, J.C.; Sneed, S.R.; Folberg, R.; Coonan, P.; Pulido, J.S. Early retinal adhesion from laser photocoagulation. *Ophthalmology* **1989**, *96*, 1523–1525. [CrossRef]
18. Zaidi, A.A.; Alvarado, R.; Irvine, A. Pneumatic retinopexy: Success rate and complications. *Br. J. Ophthalmol.* **2006**, *90*, 427–428. [CrossRef]
19. Day, S.; Grossman, D.S.; Mruthyunjaya, P.; Sloan, F.A.; Lee, P.P. One-year outcomes after retinal detachment surgery among medicare beneficiaries. *Am. J. Ophthalmol.* **2010**, *150*, 338–345. [CrossRef]
20. Chen, S.N.; Hwang, J.F. Treatment of rhegmatogenous retinal detachment in teenagers by pneumatic retinopexy technique. *Am. J. Ophthalmol.* **2007**, *143*, 217–221. [CrossRef]
21. Figueiredo, N.; Warder, D.C.; Muni, R.H.; Lee, W.W.; Yong, S.O.; Kertes, P.J. Pneumatic retinopexy as a treatment for rhegmatogenous retinal detachment in pediatric patients meeting PIVOT criteria. *Can. J. Ophthalmol.* **2022**, *57*, 359–363. [CrossRef] [PubMed]
22. Tornambe, P.E.; Hilton, G.F. Pneumatic retinopexy. A multicenter randomized controlled clinical trial comparing pneumatic retinopexy with scleral buckling. The Retinal Detachment Study Group. *Ophthalmology* **1989**, *96*, 772–783. [CrossRef] [PubMed]

23. Purtskhvanidze, K.; Hillenkamp, J.; Tode, J.; Junge, O.; Hedderich, J.; Roider, J.; Treumer, F. Thinning of inner retinal layers after vitrectomy with silicone oil versus gas endotamponade in eyes with macula-off retinal detachment. *Ophthalmologica* **2017**, *238*, 124–132. [CrossRef] [PubMed]
24. Maqsood, S.; Elalfy, M.; Abdou Hannon, A.; Hegazy, S.M.; Elborgy, E.S. Functional and structural outcomes at the foveal avascular zone with optical coherence tomography following macula off retinal detachment repair. *Clin. Ophthalmol.* **2020**, *14*, 3261–3270. [CrossRef]
25. Kaderli, S.T.; Karalezli, A.; Sul, S. Microvascular retinal alterations in rhegmatogenous retinal detachment after pneumatic retinopexy. *Acta Ophthalmol.* **2021**, *99*, 383–389. [CrossRef]
26. Muni, R.H.; Felfeli, T.; Sadda, S.R.; Juncal, V.R.; Francisconi, C.L.M.; Nittala, M.G.; Lindenberg, S.; Gunnemann, F.; Berger, A.R.; Wong, D.T.; et al. Postoperative photoreceptor integrity following pneumatic retinopexy vs pars plana vitrectomy for retinal detachment repair: A post hoc optical coherence tomography analysis from the Pneumatic Retinopexy Versus Vitrectomy for the Management of Primary Rhegmatogenous Retinal Detachment Outcomes Randomized Trial. *JAMA Ophthalmol.* **2021**, *139*, 620–627.

Journal of *Personalized Medicine*

MDPI

Article

Analysis of Retinal Microstructure in Eyes with Dissociated Optic Nerve Fiber Layer (DONFL) Appearance following Idiopathic Macular Hole Surgery: An Optical Coherence Tomography Study

Shucheng He [1,†], Xin Ye [1,*,†], Wangli Qiu [1], Shangchao Yang [1], Xiaxing Zhong [1], Yiqi Chen [2], Rui He [3] and Lijun Shen [1,2,*]

1 National Clinical Research Center for Ocular Diseases, Eye Hospital, Wenzhou Medical University, Wenzhou 325027, China
2 Department of Ophthalmology, Zhejiang Provincial People's Hospital, Hangzhou 310014, China
3 Computer Science & Software School, Hangzhou Dianzi University, Hangzhou 310018, China
* Correspondence: yexinsarah@163.com (X.Y.); ljshenysg@163.com (L.S.)
† These authors contributed equally to this work.

Abstract: (1) Purpose: This study aimed to evaluate morphological changes of the retina in eyes with dissociated optic nerve fiber layer (DONFL) appearance following internal limiting membrane (ILM) peeling for full-thickness idiopathic macular hole (IMH) on spectral-domain optical coherence tomography (SD-OCT). (2) Methods: We retrospectively analyzed 39 eyes of 39 patients with type 1 macular hole closure after a vitrectomy with ILM peeling procedure at a six-month minimum postoperative follow-up. The retinal thickness maps and cross-sectional OCT images were obtained from a clinical OCT device. The cross-sectional area of the retinal nerve fiber layer (RNFL) on cross-sectional OCT images was manually measured by ImageJ software. (3) Results: The inner retinal layers (IRLs) thickness thinned down much more in the temporal quadrant than in nasal quadrants at 2 and 6 months postoperatively ($p < 0.001$). However, the cross-sectional area of the RNFL did not change significantly at 2 and 6 months postoperatively ($p > 0.05$) when compared to preoperative data. In addition, the thinning of the IRL did not correlate with the best-corrected visual acuity (BCVA) at 6 months postoperatively. (4) Conclusions: The thickness of the IRL decreased in eyes with a DONFL appearance after ILM peeling for IMH. The thickness of the IRL decreased more in the temporal retina than in the nasal retina, but the change did not affect BCVA during the 6 months after surgery.

Keywords: dissociated optic nerve fiber layer; retinal dimples; internal limiting membrane; idiopathic full-thickness macular hole; optical coherence tomography

Citation: He, S.; Ye, X.; Qiu, W.; Yang, S.; Zhong, X.; Chen, Y.; He, R.; Shen, L. Analysis of Retinal Microstructure in Eyes with Dissociated Optic Nerve Fiber Layer (DONFL) Appearance following Idiopathic Macular Hole Surgery: An Optical Coherence Tomography Study. *J. Pers. Med.* **2023**, *13*, 255. https://doi.org/10.3390/jpm13020255

Academic Editors: Kai Jin, Chun Zhang and Yousif Subhi

Received: 27 December 2022
Revised: 21 January 2023
Accepted: 28 January 2023
Published: 30 January 2023

1. Introduction

Idiopathic macular hole (IMH) is a retinal disease that seriously threatens patients' vision and quality of life [1,2]. The mechanism of IMH involves the disruption or loss of the Müller cell cone in the fovea, and this is caused by the vitreoretinal traction perifovea [3–5] (see Figure 1C). A vitrectomy with the internal limiting membrane (ILM) peeling procedure has been proven to promote postoperative macular hole closure and improve visual function in previous studies [6,7]. However, ILM plays an important role in homeostasis and maintenance of inner retinal layers, as it is the basal membrane of Müller cells. Moreover, in some cases, the removal of the ILM results in various complications, such as swelling of the arcuate retinal nerve fiber layer (SANFL), macular retinal displacement, dissociated optical nerve fiber layer (DONFL), etc. [8]. The study on the morphological changes of the retina after the removal of the ILM in eyes with macular hole can help us to further elucidate the potential damage caused by the surgery.

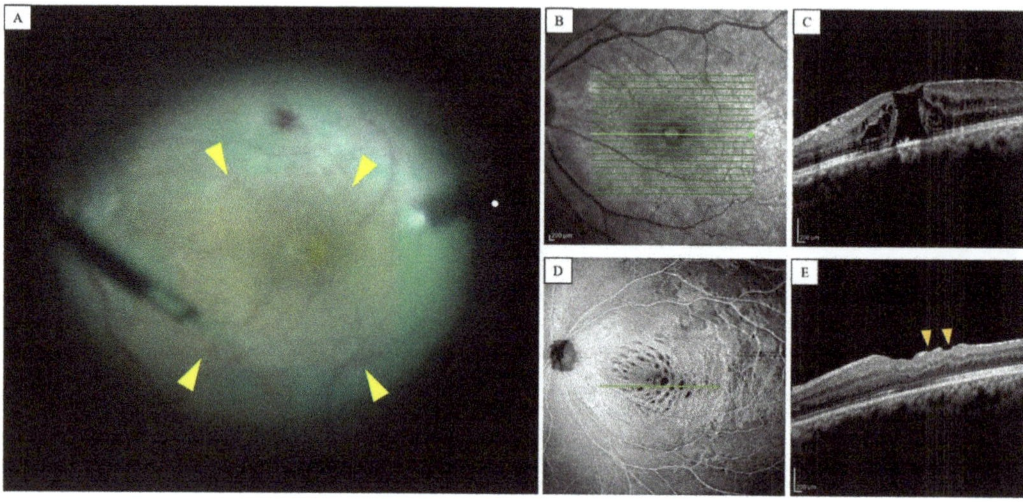

Figure 1. Left eye of a 61-year-old man treated with vitrectomy and ILM peeling for IMH. (**A**). The ILM around the macular hole was removed using pinch-and-peel technique after indocyanine green staining. The yellow arrows represent the extent of the inner limiting membrane peeling. A full-thickness macular hole was observed in fundus image (**B**) and OCT B-scan (**C**) before the surgery. The green line with the arrow in (**B**) indicates the scan line for the B-scan OCT images in (**C**). En face OCT images (**D**) at four-month postoperatively showed a clear CMDS appearance (i.e., concentric dark spots) inside the ILM peeling area. And some focal dimples corresponding to dark spots on green line in (**D**), were visible in the RNFL on B-scan OCT images in (**E**) (yellow arrows).

Optical coherence tomography (OCT) is a non-invasive optical imaging technique that enables in vivo imaging of the structural morphology and blood flow (OCT angiography) of the retina in both human and a variety of veterinary species [9,10]. DONFL appears as dimples (see Figure 1E) in the inner retinal layers on cross-sectional OCT images and as concentric macular dark spots (CMDS) in en face OCT images [8,11] (see Figure 1D). Several studies have shown that a DONFL appearance occurs without the loss of the nerve fiber layer and argued that DONFL is caused by the rearrangement rather than the loss of optic nerve fibers after ILM peeling [12,13]. However, some scholars believe that DONFL involves damages in the deeper area under the retinal nerve fiber layer (RNFL), such as the ganglion cell layer–inner plexiform layer (GCL–IPL) complex [14,15]. To date, the pathogenesis of DONFL and the role of the retinal layer have not been well clarified.

Recently, with the help of high-resolution OCT, the structure of the retina could be analyzed layer by layer, using thickness maps. Several studies have shown that ILM peeling in IMH causes progressive thinning of some retina layers [16–18]. However, it is not known whether this retinal-layer thinning is associated with the formation of DONFL, and there is a lack of longitudinal observations of the retinal structure in DONFL patients after ILM peeling. The study of the retinal layer changes in DONFL may help to shed light on the formation mechanism of DONFL and its potential damage to vision.

Given the high incidence of DONFL after ILM peeling in IMH [19], this study aimed to evaluate the retinal structure in eyes with DONFL after ILM peeling for IMH through long-term follow-up to explore the mechanism of DONFL formation. We also analyzed the correlation between the change of retinal layers and visual acuity after surgery. We hope this study can help to provide more information for clinical practice to improve the surgical procedures.

2. Methods

2.1. Ethical Approval

This was a retrospective study that adhered to the tenets of the Declaration of Helsinki. Institutional Review Board (IRB) approval was obtained from the Affiliated Eye Hospital of Wenzhou Medical University, and informed consent was obtained from all subjects.

2.2. Inclusion and Exclusion Criteria

Inclusion criteria were eyes diagnosed as IMH and underwent ILM peeling between January 2017 and September 2020. All the included eyes achieved a type 1 closure pattern and at least 6 months of postoperative follow-up. The type 1 closure of IMH was defined as some reconstitution of the banded anatomy [20]. All the included eyes' pre- and postoperative fundus photographs, as well as OCT scans with a minimum follow-up of six months, were accessed. The size of the macular hole was measured as the minimum hole width or the narrowest aperture size in the middle retina on cross-sectional OCT images, as defined by The International Vitreomacular Traction Study (IVTS) Group on initial presentation [21]. Eyes with other severe vitreoretinal diseases (e.g., glaucoma, retinitis pigmentosa, diabetic retinopathy, and pathological myopia), a history of the previous vitrectomy, and poor OCT image quality were excluded from the study.

2.3. Surgical Procedure

The standard three-port pars plana vitrectomies were performed in all patients by a surgeon, using a 23-gauge transconjunctival vitrectomy system (see Figure 1A). Phacoemulsification with intraocular lens implantation would be performed if the cataract was severe enough to interfere with intraocular surgery. Triamcinolone acetonide was used to assist posterior vitreous detachment (PVD). ILM was removed around the macular hole in 2–3 disc diameters, using a pinch-and-peel technique with forceps stained with 0.02 mL of indocyanine green (0.025 mg/mL) (see Figure 1A). Sterile air was filled in the vitreous cavity following the exchange of gas and liquid. For a minimum of seven days after surgery, all patients had to remain facedown.

2.4. Data Collection

Information collected included demographic data (e.g., age and sex), laterality, pre- and postoperative best-corrected visual acuity (BCVA), lens status, B-scan SD-OCT images (Spectralis HRA, Heidelberg Engineering, Germany), and en face OCT images (RTVue, Optovue, San Francisco, CA, USA). The B-scan mode included a linear horizontal scan of $20^\circ \times 15^\circ$ (6.6*4.9 mm). BCVA measurements were performed by using the Snellen chart and were converted to units of logarithms of the minimum angle of resolution (logMAR) for statistical analyses. The postoperative parameters were analyzed two and six months after surgery.

On en face OCT images, all postoperative images were assessed to determine whether or not inner retinal dimples were present. The retinal layers were automated segmented with the 6*6 mm scan mode in the macular region, using the RTVue XR OCT. One retinal specialist would make manual adjustments if the segmentation was improper before further retinal thickness measurement. Then the mean thickness of the total retinal layer (TRL), the outer retinal layer (ORL), and the inner retinal layer (IRL) of the parafoveal area (i.e., the area with an inner diameter of 1mm and an outer diameter of 3 mm) were automated measured with embed software and exported for further analysis (see Figure 2). TRL was defined as the retina layer between the ILM and the retinal pigment epithelium (RPE), the ORL was defined as the retina layer from the inner nuclear layer to the RPE, and the IRL was defined as the retina layer from the ILM to the inner plexiform layer. All the thickness data in each quadrant were exported for further analysis. In addition, the ImageJ (software version 1.52; National Institutes of Health, Bethesda, MD, USA) was used to quantitatively assess the cross-sectional area of the RNFL. This measurement method has been proven effective in previous studies [13]. In brief, three horizontal B-scan OCT images (i.e., subfoveal, the closest superior, and inferior to the fovea) with 6 mm scan length and 0.25 mm intervals at each follow-up visit were selected. The area of RNFL in each image was measured manually, using the ImageJ program by one observer, and the area was quantified in pixels (see Figure 2). Fifty OCT images were chosen randomly from the collected images to determine the reproducibility of the measurement, and two observers were asked to evaluate them individually. To determine the repeatability of the measurement, Observer 1 was asked to measure the same 50 images one week after the first measurement and was blind to the previous scores.

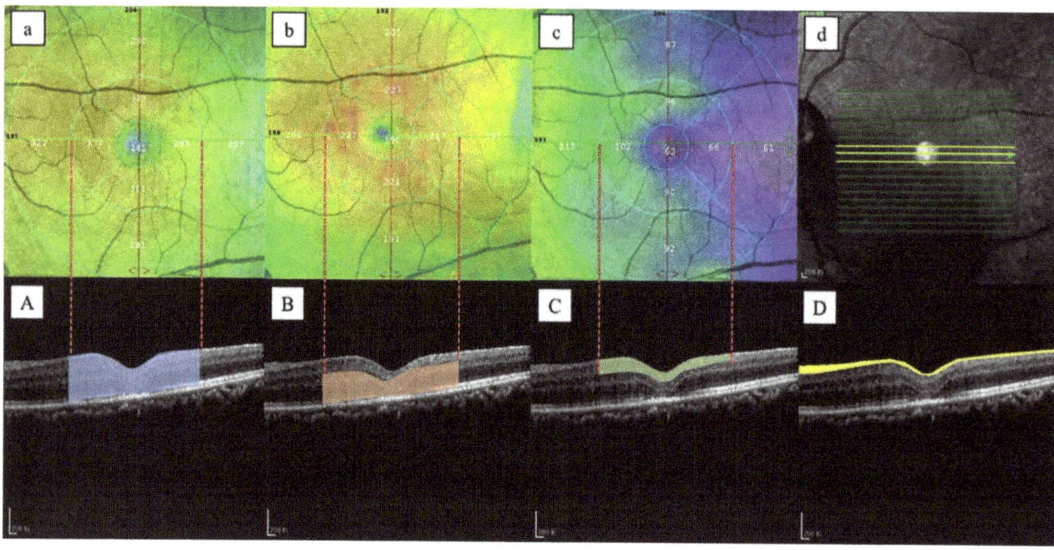

Figure 2. Left eye of a 57-year-old woman treated with vitrectomy and ILM peeling for IMH. (**a**–**c**). The thickness of TRL, ORL, and IRL in different parafoveal regions was automatically identified using the Early Treatment Diabetic Retinopathy Study (ETDRS) grid and measured by RTVue XR OCT. (**d**). The B-scan OCT images of the fovea, the closest superior to the fovea, and the closest inferior to the fovea were used for the measurement of RNFL cross-sectional area. (**A**). The TRL was defined as the area between the ILM and the RPE as the area shown in blue. (**B**). The ORL was defined as the area from the inner nuclear layer to the RPE as the area shown in orange. (**C**). The IRL was defined as the area from the ILM to the inner plexiform layer as the area shown in green. (**D**). RNFL cross-sectional area (i.e., yellow section) in B-scan OCT images was measured manually using ImageJ software.

2.5. Statistical Analysis

Statistical analyses were conducted with statistics software (IBM SPSS, version 26; IBM Corp., Armonk, NY, USA). The normality of data distribution was confirmed by using the Shapiro–Wilk test. The normally distributed variables were expressed as mean ± standard deviation, and the non-normally distributed variables were expressed as median (interquartile range). Repeated measures ANOVA was used to evaluate the changes in different retinal layers over time. Considering inter-group correlations, generalized estimating equations (GEEs) were used to analyze differences in the reduction of retinal layer thickness in different quadrants. Multiple comparisons between the groups within each analysis were performed by using the Bonferroni correction test. Correlation tests were conducted by using Spearman's correlation test. A p-value of less than 0.05 was considered statistically significant.

3. Results

3.1. Subject Characteristics and Incidence of DONFL

The study included 39 eyes from 39 patients with at least a 6-month follow-up (9 men and 30 women, ages 25 to 84, mean age, 59.487 ± 10.406 years). The axial length was, on average, 24.318 ± 1.914 mm. Except for the eye of a 24-year-old woman who had no diagnosis of cataract, all of the included eyes underwent phacoemulsification and intraocular lens implantation. In total, there were 8 (20.51%) eyes with a small macular hole, 8 (20.51%) eyes with a median macular hole, and 23 (58.97%) eyes with a large macular hole. Mean preoperative BCVA was 0.929 ± 0.494 logMAR units, and BCVA 6 months postoperatively was 0.311 ± 0.283 logMAR units. The improvement in BCVA from the baseline was statistically significant ($p < 0.001$). At the initial checkup two months following surgery, 30 eyes (76.92%) had DONFL in all four quadrants, compared to 9 eyes (23.08%) that had DONFL exclusively in the temporal quadrant. DONFL was noticed throughout the course after 6 months following surgery in each of the four quadrants (100%). Table 1 gives all the information.

Table 1. Demographics and clinical characteristics of study subjects (n = 41).

Variables	Value
Age (years, mean ± SD)	59.487 ± 10.406
Gender (N, %)	
Male	9, 23.08%
Female	30, 76.92%
Eyes (N, %)	
Right	18, 46.15%
Left	21, 53.85%
AL (mm, mean ± SD)	24.318 ± 1.914
BCVA (logMAR, mean ± SD)	
Preoperative	0.929 ± 0.494
2 months postoperative	0.415 ± 0.294
6 months postoperative	0.311 ± 0.283
Classification of IMH	
Small (N, %)	8 (20.51%)
Medium (N, %)	8 (20.51%)
Large (N, %)	23 (58.97%)

AL, axial length; BCVA, best correct visual acuity.

3.2. Retinal Thickness Decreased in DONFL after Surgery

The retinal thickness analysis was performed in all eyes. The mean thickness of the layers for each quadrant during the follow-up is listed in Supplementary Table S2. The trends of retinal thickness in each quadrant are shown in Figure 3. The thickness of TRL and ORL in all quadrants was decreased at the 6-month postoperative follow-up ($p < 0.001$). Moreover, the IRL thickness in all quadrants decreased at 6-month postoperative follow-up ($p < 0.001$ for temporal, superior, and inferior; $p = 0.008$ for nasal). The cross-sectional area of the RNFL increased slightly from 2945.436 ± 559.580 pixels preoperatively to 3048.222 ± 572.067 pixels at 2 months postoperatively, but the change was not statistically significant ($p = 0.623$). Four months later, the cross-sectional area of the RNFL later decreased to 2841.256 ± 590.553 pixels at 6 months postoperatively ($p = 0.044$), but the finding was not statistically different from the baseline ($p = 0.463$) (as shown in Figure 3). The intraclass correlation coefficient (ICC) of the measurements for intra-observer repeatability and inter-observer reproducibility were, respectively, 0.971 and 0.960. The results of the Bland–Altman analysis showed that the measurements had good intra-observer repeatability and inter-observer reproducibility (as shown in Figure 4). The intervals between the 95% limits of agreement were relatively small and suitable for clinical evaluation (inter-observer, −218.7 to 348.5; intra-observer, −240.0 to 403.5). This suggests that the RNFL area measurement is generally accurate and trustworthy.

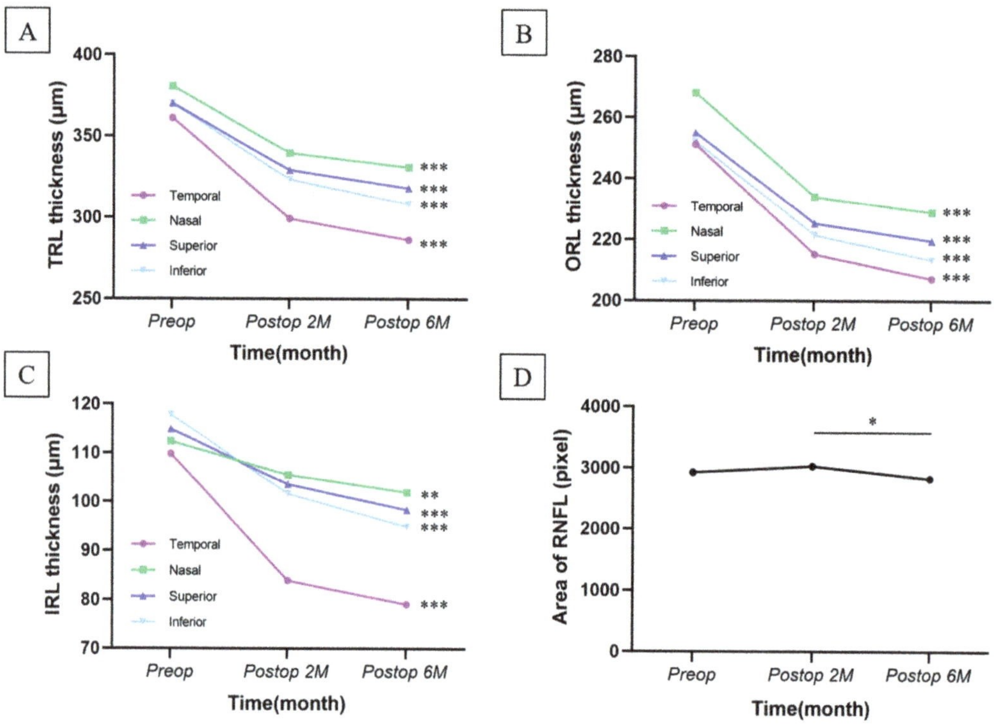

Figure 3. Trends of changes and regional differences in the different retinal layers of the patients with DONFL during postoperative follow-up. (**A**–**C**). The thickness of TRL, ORL, and IRL decreased significantly in all quadrants. (**D**). The area of RNFL increased slightly at 2-month operatively with no significant difference, then decreased significantly between 2 months operatively and 6 months operatively, but there is still no significant difference compared to the preoperative. * Statistically significant difference($p < 0.05$). ** Statistically significant difference($p < 0.01$). *** Statistically significant difference($p < 0.001$).

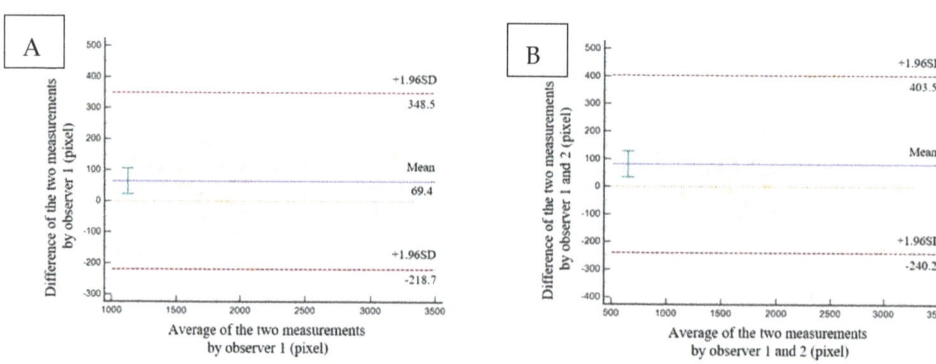

Figure 4. Results of intra-observer and inter-observer agreement for RNFL measurement. (**A**) Results of intra-observer agreement for RNFL measurement. The abscissa was the average of the two measurements from observer 1, and the ordinate was the difference of the two measurements from the same observer. (**B**) Results of inter-observer agreement for RNFL measurement. The abscissa was the average of the two measurements from observer 1 and observer 2, and the ordinate was the difference between the two measurements from observer 1 and observer 2.

3.3. The Extent of Thinning in the Layers of the Retina

We further compared the extent of thinning in ORL and IRL in each quadrant during the 6-month follow-ups (Table 2). The result showed that there was no significant difference in the reduction of ORL thickness between the temporal and nasal quadrants at the 2- and 6-month follow-ups ($p = 1.000$). There was also no significant difference in the reduction of ORL thickness between the superior and inferior quadrants at the 2- and 6-month follow-ups ($p = 1.000$). At the 2- and 6-month follow-ups, it was discovered that the IRL thickness decreased more in the temporal quadrant than in the nasal quadrants, and the differences were statistically significant ($p < 0.001$). However, no statistical difference was found between superior and inferior quadrants in IRL thickness decrease ($p = 0.171$ for 2 months, $p = 0.077$ for 6 months). The retinal thickness at baseline was analyzed, and the result (Supplementary Table S3) showed that the nasal ORL was significantly thicker than the temporal ORL ($p < 0.001$). However, there was also no significant difference between the superior and inferior ORL thickness ($p = 1.000$). As for IRL, the temporal IRL was thinner than the nasal IRL, but there was no significant difference ($p = 1.000$). The thickness of superior IRL and inferior IRL also showed no difference ($p = 1.000$).

Table 2. Reduction of inner and outer retinal thickness in each quadrant in the patients with DONFL during the different postoperative periods.

	Temporal	Nasal	*p1*	Superior	Inferior	*p2*
ORL						
2 months	28 (−1, 54)	32 (−3, 56)	1.000	20 (0, 46)	23 (−3, 58)	1.000
6 months	34 (11, 67)	35 (0, 57)	1.000	25 (6, 50)	33 (2, 57)	1.000
IRL						
2 months	22 (14, 32)	7 (−6, 20)	< 0.001 †	11 (0, 21)	13 (−1, 25)	0.171
6 months	25 (18, 37)	10 (−1, 25)	< 0.001 †	17 (3, 27)	17 (5, 29)	0.077

DONFL, dissociated optic nerve fiber layer; ORL, outer retinal layer; IRL, inner retinal layer. The *p1* was obtained by Bonferroni correct test comparing the data of temporal and nasal in GEE analysis, and *p2* was obtained by Bonferroni correct test comparing the data of superior and inferior in GEE analysis.

3.4. Correlation between Retinal Layers Thinning and BCVA

In order to further explore whether the thinning in the IRL and ORL was correlated with the postoperative BCVA in eyes with DONFL, we analyzed the correlation between the extent of thinning in both layers and BCVA 6 months after surgery, using the Spearman correlation test. The results indicated that BCVA did not correlate with IRL or ORL thinning in each quadrant (Table 3) and also did not correlate with the mean thinning of IRL or ORL.

Table 3. The correlation between BCVA and the reduction of retinal thickness in each quadrant in the patients with DONFL 6 months after surgery, using Spearman's correlation test.

	Temporal	Nasal	Superior	Inferior	Mean
Outer retina layer					
***r*-value**	0.161	0.14	0.071	0.045	0.093
***p*-value**	0.328	0.394	0.666	0.786	0.575
Inner retina layer					
***r*-value**	-0.063	0.104	0.038	0.103	0.069
***p*-value**	0.704	0.529	0.816	0.534	0.678

4. Discussion

Previous studies have shown a strong link between ILM peeling and the formation of DONFL [14,22,23]. Mitamura et al. [12] found that DONFL was present in 62.2% of the ILM peeling group limited in areas with ILM peeling and 0.0% in the non-ILM peeling group. Another study reported that the incidence of DONFL was as high as 100% after idiopathic full-thickness macular hole (FTMH) surgery [11]. Most studies consider defects in the IRL in DONFL after ILM peeling to be limited to RNFL changes and consider DONFL to be a reorganization of RNFL. However, some research argued that DONFL involves damages in IRL rather than RNFL rearrangement only [14].

In this study, we analyzed 39 of 39 DONFL eyes and found significant reductions in ORL and IRL thickness in all quadrants at 6 months postoperatively. A further analysis showed that the thickness of the temporal IRL decreased more than the IRL thickness in the nasal quadrant; these findings are similar to the findings of other researchers. For example, Tada et al. [18], by using retinal thickness maps, found that ILM peeling resulted in progressive thinning of the temporal inner retina at 6 months postoperatively, but no significant changes were found in the nasal inner retina. In addition, the distribution pattern of changes in IRL thickness is highly similar to what we have in our previous quantitative study of DONFL: the severity of DONFL was greater on the temporal side than in the other quadrants [24]. Given that DONFL is an inner retinal appearance and that the distribution of changes in ORL did not have a similar pattern to that of DONFL, we speculate that the formation of DONFL might be related to a reduction in IRL thickness. As an indirect indicator of retinal depression, the cross-sectional area of RNFL, compared to preoperative data, increased within 2 months postoperatively and decreased at 6 months postoperatively, yet these changes did not reach statistical significance. These changes in the RNFL were also observed by Clark et al. [25]; the study found swelling of the inner retina within 1 week to 1 month after ILM peeling. Using intraoperative OCT, Runkel et al. [19] found an increase in intraoperative nerve fiber layer thickness and a significant association with the development of postoperative DONFL appearance. Generally, the nerve fiber layer swelling disappeared after an average of 2 months postoperatively, so the reduction in RNFL cross-sectional area observed in this study between 2 and 6 months after surgery may be related to the disappearance of swelling, and the RNFL may be rearranged rather than becoming defective in the development of DONFL.

Given that the RNFL area did not alter considerably in our investigation, a drop in IRL thickness would have happened in deeper layers, such as GCL–IPL, after ILM peeling. Demirel et al. [15] also discovered that, following ILM peeling, the GCL–IPL thickness decreased, and the GCL thinning was particularly noticeable in the inner retinal dimples. According to researchers, retinal ganglion cell (RGC) mortality may not be the source of GCL thinning in the foveal region since, if RGC death resulted in the emergence of DONFL, there should be a corresponding arcuate loss of nerve fibers and a visual-field deficiency. However, previous studies have not observed any visual-field defects in DONFL patients [22]. Therefore, the thinning of GCL in the depressed area may be related to the loss or damage of Müller cells in this area [26]. The endfeet of Müller cells participated in the formation of the ILM [27]. Stripping the ILM may deprive the Müller cells of their endfeet function, causing the remainder to degenerate.

Another hypothesis in the pathogenesis of DONFL is related to anoikis in RGCs [28]. Anchorage-dependent cells that undergo dissociation from the surrounding extracellular matrix experience a type of apoptosis known as anoikis [29]. As we all know, ILMs are formed by the foot processes of Müller cells, and the expression of integrins has been detected in the ILM [30]. Moreover, since the focal adhesion kinase is expressed in RGCs [31,32], RGCs might act as an anchorage-dependent cell adjacent to the ILM, and ILM peeling might trigger the anoikis in RGCs. Recent studies have suggested that there may be undifferentiated cells in the fovea, such as retinal stem cells [33]. This sets the foundation for apoptosis, as apoptosis occurs in a large number of cells during the integration of early generated neurons [34,35]. It has been shown that ganglion cells express E-cadherin during embryogenesis [36], and E-cadherin is known to be a glycoprotein associated with anoikis. βA3/A1 crystallin, a protein associated with apoptosis, has also been discovered [37]. RGCs instead of Müller cells expresses the protein. Therefore, we speculate that the appearance of DONFL is due to ILM-peeling-induced anoikis in newly formed RGCs from retinal stem cells rather than in Müller cells. Apoptosis of these newly formed RGCs promotes a DONFL appearance and leads to a reduction in IRL thickness. In the present study, there was no correlation between IRL changes in each quadrant and postoperative BCVA

6 months after surgery. This finding can be explained by the above theory because the newly generated RGCs may not yet be integrated into the neural network and are not involved in visual function. Moreover, the cross-sectional area of RNFL did not change compared to preoperative data, and this serves as another piece of evidence for the above theory. The reason for the greater reduction in retinal thickness in the temporal IRL may be that the nerve-fiber layer is thinner on the temporal side than other sides, and the ganglion cells are less protected by RNFL, thereby leaving the area more susceptible to damages. Based on these explanations, we propose that developmental changes in DONFL may be attributed to multiple factors, such as RNFL layer rearrangements and GCL–IPL layer defects, and are closely associated with alterations in Müller cells and RGCs.

The main limitations of this study are listed as follows: (1) This study was retrospective, and the sample size of patients was relatively small. (2) The detection of visual function is relatively simple and lacks more evaluation of visual function except for BCVA. (3) This was a single-center study, and a multicentric study is necessary for further analysis.

In conclusion, there was thinning in IRL and ORL in patients with DONFL, and the IRL thinning mainly involved the temporal retina. The results show that there is no significant correlation between retinal thinning and postoperative BCVA in DONFL patients.

Supplementary Materials: The following supporting information can be downloaded at: https://www.mdpi.com/article/10.3390/jpm13020255/s1, Table S1: The area of RNFL in the patients with DONFL during postoperative follow-up; Table S2: The retinal thickness of each layer in each quadrant in the patients with DONFL during postoperative follow-up; Table S3: The baseline of inner and outer retinal thickness in each quadrant in the patients with DONFL.

Author Contributions: L.S. had full access to all the data in the study and will take responsibility for the integrity of the data and the accuracy of the data analysis. Study concept and design: S.H. and X.Y. Acquisition, analysis, or interpretation of data: S.H. and X.Y.. Drafting of the manuscript: S.H., X.Y., W.Q., X.Z., S.Y. and R.H. Critical revision of the manuscript for important intellectual content: L.S. Study supervision: L.S., X.Y. and Y.C. All authors have read and agreed to the published version of the manuscript.

Funding: This work was supported in part by the Medical Science and Technology Project of Zhejiang Province (No. 2023KY915).

Institutional Review Board Statement: The study was conducted in accordance with the Declaration of Helsinki and approved by the Institutional Review Board of Affiliated Eye Hospital of Wenzhou Medical University (H2022-012-K-12-001).

Informed Consent Statement: Informed consent was obtained from all subjects involved in the study.

Data Availability Statement: The datasets used and analyzed during the current study are available from the corresponding author upon reasonable request.

Acknowledgments: The authors acknowledge Vicky Chung.

Conflicts of Interest: The authors declare no conflict of interest.

References

1. Gass, J.D. Idiopathic senile macular hole. Its early stages and pathogenesis. *Arch. Ophthalmol.* **1988**, *106*, 629–639. [CrossRef] [PubMed]
2. Cheong, K.X.; Xu, L.; Ohno-Matsui, K.; Sabanayagam, C.; Saw, S.M.; Hoang, Q.V. An evidence-based review of the epidemiology of myopic traction maculopathy. *Surv. Ophthalmol.* **2022**, *67*, 1603–1630. [CrossRef] [PubMed]
3. Gass, J.D. Müller cell cone, an overlooked part of the anatomy of the fovea centralis: Hypotheses concerning its role in the pathogenesis of macular hole and foveomacualr retinoschisis. *Arch. Ophthalmol.* **1999**, *117*, 821–823. [CrossRef] [PubMed]
4. Bikbova, G.; Oshitari, T.; Baba, T.; Yamamoto, S.; Mori, K. Pathogenesis and Management of Macular Hole: Review of Current Advances. *J. Ophthalmol.* **2019**, *2019*, 3467381. [CrossRef]
5. Bringmann, A.; Unterlauft, J.D.; Barth, T.; Wiedemann, R.; Rehak, M.; Wiedemann, P. Müller cells and astrocytes in tractional macular disorders. *Prog. Retin. Eye Res.* **2022**, *86*, 100977. [CrossRef]
6. Wendel, R.T.; Patel, A.C.; Kelly, N.E.; Salzano, T.C.; Wells, J.W.; Novack, G.D. Vitreous surgery for macular holes. *Ophthalmology* **1993**, *100*, 1671–1676. [CrossRef]

7. Tao, J.; Chen, H.; Chen, Y.; Yu, J.; Xu, J.; Mao, J.; Lin, L.; Shen, L. Efficacy of air tamponade treatment of idiopathic macular holes of different diameters and of follow-up intravitreal air tamponade for persistent holes. *Retina* **2022**, *42*, 877–882. [CrossRef]
8. Tadayoni, R.; Paques, M.; Massin, P.; Mouki-Benani, S.; Mikol, J.; Gaudric, A. Dissociated optic nerve fiber layer appearance of the fundus after idiopathic epiretinal membrane removal. *Ophthalmology* **2001**, *108*, 2279–2283. [CrossRef]
9. Meleppat, R.K.; Fortenbach, C.R.; Jian, Y.; Martinez, E.S.; Wagner, K.; Modjtahedi, B.S.; Motta, M.J.; Ramamurthy, D.L.; Schwab, I.R.; Zawadzki, R.J. In Vivo Imaging of Retinal and Choroidal Morphology and Vascular Plexuses of Vertebrates Using Swept-Source Optical Coherence Tomography. *Transl. Vis. Sci. Technol.* **2022**, *11*, 11. [CrossRef]
10. Meleppat, R.K.; Zhang, P.; Ju, M.J.; Manna, S.K.; Jian, Y.; Pugh, E.N.; Zawadzki, R.J. Directional optical coherence tomography reveals melanin concentration-dependent scattering properties of retinal pigment epithelium. *J. Biomed. Opt.* **2019**, *24*, 066011. [CrossRef]
11. Alkabes, M.; Salinas, C.; Vitale, L.; Burés-Jelstrup, A.; Nucci, P.; Mateo, C. En face optical coherence tomography of inner retinal defects after internal limiting membrane peeling for idiopathic macular hole. *Investig. Ophthalmol. Vis. Sci.* **2011**, *52*, 8349–8355. [CrossRef] [PubMed]
12. Mitamura, Y.; Ohtsuka, K. Relationship of dissociated optic nerve fiber layer appearance to internal limiting membrane peeling. *Ophthalmology* **2005**, *112*, 1766–1770. [CrossRef] [PubMed]
13. Kim, Y.J.; Lee, K.S.; Joe, S.G.; Kim, J.-G. Incidence and quantitative analysis of dissociated optic nerve fiber layer appearance: Real loss of retinal nerve fiber layer? *Eur. J. Ophthalmol.* **2018**, *28*, 317–323. [CrossRef]
14. Nukada, K.; Hangai, M.; Ooto, S.; Yoshikawa, M.; Yoshimura, N. Tomographic features of macula after successful macular hole surgery. *Investig. Ophthalmol. Vis. Sci.* **2013**, *54*, 2417–2428. [CrossRef]
15. Demirel, S.; Abdullayev, A.; Yanık, Ö.; Batıoğlu, F.; Özmert, E. Evaluation of Ganglion Cell-Inner Plexiform Layer Thickness after Vitreoretinal Surgery with Internal Limiting Membrane Peeling in Cases with Idiopathic Macular Hole. *Turk. J. Ophthalmol.* **2017**, *47*, 138–143. [CrossRef] [PubMed]
16. Ohta, K.; Sato, A.; Fukui, E. Retinal thickness in eyes with idiopathic macular hole after vitrectomy with internal limiting membrane peeling. *Graefes Arch. Clin. Exp. Ophthalmol.* **2013**, *251*, 1273–1279. [CrossRef] [PubMed]
17. Faria, M.Y.; Ferreira, N.P.; Cristóvao, D.M.; Mano, S.; Sousa, D.C.; Monteiro-Grillo, M. Tomographic Structural Changes of Retinal Layers after Internal Limiting Membrane Peeling for Macular Hole Surgery. *Ophthalmic Res.* **2018**, *59*, 24–29. [CrossRef] [PubMed]
18. Tada, A.; Machida, S.; Hara, Y.; Ebihara, S.; Ishizuka, M.; Gonmori, M. Long-Term Observations of Thickness Changes of Each Retinal Layer following Macular Hole Surgery. *J. Ophthalmol.* **2021**, *2021*, 4624164. [CrossRef]
19. Runkle, A.P.; Srivastava, S.K.; Yuan, A.; Kaiser, P.K.; Singh, R.P.; Reese, J.L.; Ehlers, J.P. Factors associated with development of dissociated optic nerve fiber layer appearance in the pioneer intraoperative optical coherence tomography study. *Retina* **2018**, *38* (Suppl. 1), S103–S109. [CrossRef]
20. Rossi, T.; Bacherini, D.; Caporossi, T.; Telani, S.; Iannetta, D.; Rizzo, S.; Moysidis, S.N.; Koulisis, N.; Mahmoud, T.H.; Ripandelli, G. Macular hole closure patterns: An updated classification. *Graefes Arch. Clin. Exp. Ophthalmol.* **2020**, *258*, 2629–2638. [CrossRef]
21. Duker, J.S.; Kaiser, P.K.; Binder, S.; de Smet, M.D.; Gaudric, A.; Reichel, E.; Sadda, S.R.; Sebag, J.; Spaide, R.F.; Stalmans, P. The International Vitreomacular Traction Study Group classification of vitreomacular adhesion, traction, and macular hole. *Ophthalmology* **2013**, *120*, 2611–2619. [CrossRef] [PubMed]
22. Ito, Y.; Terasaki, H.; Takahashi, A.; Yamakoshi, T.; Kondo, M.; Nakamura, M. Dissociated optic nerve fiber layer appearance after internal limiting membrane peeling for idiopathic macular holes. *Ophthalmology* **2005**, *112*, 1415–1420. [CrossRef] [PubMed]
23. Kumar, V.; Dubey, D.; Kumawat, D.; Markan, A.; Chandra, P.; Chandra, M.; Kumar, A. Role of internal limiting membrane peeling in the prevention of epiretinal membrane formation following vitrectomy for retinal detachment: A randomised trial. *Br. J. Ophthalmol.* **2020**, *104*, 1271–1276. [CrossRef]
24. Ye, X.; Xu, J.; He, S.; Wang, J.; Yang, J.; Tao, J.; Chen, Y.; Shen, L. Quantitative evaluation of dissociated optic nerve fibre layer (DONFL) following idiopathic macular hole surgery. *Eye* 2022. [CrossRef]
25. Clark, A.; Balducci, N.; Pichi, F.; Veronese, C.; Morara, M.; Torrazza, C.; Ciardella, A.P. Swelling of the arcuate nerve fiber layer after internal limiting membrane peeling. *Retina* **2012**, *32*, 1608–1613. [CrossRef] [PubMed]
26. Spaide, R.F. "Dissociated optic nerve fiber layer appearance" after internal limiting membrane removal is inner retinal dimpling. *Retina* **2012**, *32*, 1719–1726. [CrossRef]
27. Vecino, E.; Rodriguez, F.D.; Ruzafa, N.; Pereiro, X.; Sharma, S.C. Glia-neuron interactions in the mammalian retina. *Prog Retin Eye Res.* **2016**, *51*, 1–40. [CrossRef]
28. Ikeda, T.; Nakamura, K.; Sato, T.; Kida, T.; Oku, H. Involvement of Anoikis in Dissociated Optic Nerve Fiber Layer Appearance. *Int. J. Mol. Sci.* **2021**, *22*, 1724. [CrossRef]
29. Taddei, M.L.; Giannoni, E.; Fiaschi, T.; Chiarugi, P. Anoikis: An emerging hallmark in health and diseases. *J. Pathol.* **2012**, *226*, 380–393. [CrossRef]
30. Brem, R.B.; Robbins, S.G.; Wilson, D.J.; O'Rourke, L.M.; Mixon, R.N.; Robertson, J.E.; Planck, S.R.; Rosenbaum, J.T. Immunolocalization of integrins in the human retina. *Investig. Ophthalmol Vis. Sci.* **1994**, *35*, 3466–3474.
31. D'Onofrio, P.M.; Shabanzadeh, A.P.; Choi, B.K.; Bähr, M.; Koeberle, P.D. MMP Inhibition Preserves Integrin Ligation and FAK Activation to Induce Survival and Regeneration in RGCs Following Optic Nerve Damage. *Investig. Ophthalmol. Vis. Sci.* **2019**, *60*, 634–649. [CrossRef]

32. Li, Y.; Chen, Y.-M.; Sun, M.-M.; Guo, X.-D.; Wang, Y.-C.; Zhang, Z.-Z. Inhibition on Apoptosis Induced by Elevated Hydrostatic Pressure in Retinal Ganglion Cell-5 via Laminin Upregulating β1-integrin/Focal Adhesion Kinase/Protein Kinase B Signaling Pathway. *Chin. Med. J.* **2016**, *129*, 976–983. [CrossRef] [PubMed]
33. Saha, A.; Capowski, E.; Fernandez Zepeda, M.A.; Nelson, E.C.; Gamm, D.M.; Sinha, R. Cone photoreceptors in human stem cell-derived retinal organoids demonstrate intrinsic light responses that mimic those of primate fovea. *Cell Stem Cell* **2022**, *29*, 460–471.e3. [CrossRef] [PubMed]
34. Bunk, E.C.; König, H.G.; Bernas, T.; Engel, T.; Henshall, D.C.; Kirby, B.P.; Prehn, J.H.M. BH3-only proteins BIM and PUMA in the regulation of survival and neuronal differentiation of newly generated cells in the adult mouse hippocampus. *Cell Death Dis.* **2010**, *1*, e15. [CrossRef]
35. Lepousez, G.; Lledo, P.-M. Life and death decision in adult neurogenesis: In praise of napping. *Neuron* **2011**, *71*, 768–771. [CrossRef] [PubMed]
36. Oblander, S.A.; Ensslen-Craig, S.E.; Longo, F.M.; Brady-Kalnay, S.M. E-cadherin promotes retinal ganglion cell neurite outgrowth in a protein tyrosine phosphatase-mu-dependent manner. *Mol. Cell. Neurosci.* **2007**, *34*, 481–492. [CrossRef] [PubMed]
37. Parthasarathy, G.; Ma, B.; Zhang, C.; Gongora, C.; Samuel Zigler, J.; Duncan, M.K.; Sinha, D. Expression of βA3/A1-crystallin in the developing and adult rat eye. *J. Mol. Histol.* **2011**, *42*, 59–69. [CrossRef]

Journal of *Personalized Medicine*

MDPI

Article

A Novel *PAX6* Frameshift Mutation Identified in a Large Chinese Family with Congenital Aniridia

Chenghu Wang [1,†], Weihua Yang [2,†], Xiumiao Li [1], Chenchen Zhou [1], Jinghua Liu [1], Ling Jin [1], Qin Jiang [1,*] and Yun Wang [2,*]

1 Eye Hospital, Nanjing Medical University, Nanjing 210029, China
2 Shenzhen Eye Hospital, Shenzhen Eye Institute, Jinan University, Shenzhen 518040, China
* Correspondence: jqin710@vip.sina.com (Q.J.); s_ywang@126.com (Y.W.)
† These authors contributed to the manuscript equally.

Abstract: Congenital aniridia is a rare autosomal dominant congenital ocular disorder. Genetic studies suggest that heterozygous mutations in the developmental regulator *PAX6* gene or the related regulatory regions leading to haploinsufficiency are the main cause of congenital aniridia. In this study, the clinical characteristics and pathogenic mutation of a four-generation Chinese family with congenital aniridia were investigated. All members recruited in this study underwent comprehensive ophthalmic examinations. Targeted gene capture sequencing and Sanger sequencing were performed to screen and confirm the candidate pathogenicity gene and its mutation. A multiple alignment of homologous sequences covering the identified mutation from different species was investigated, and the mutant protein structure was predicted using Swiss-Model. Additionally, the prediction of pathogenicity was analyzed using the ACMG Guidelines. Thirteen patients in this pedigree were diagnosed with congenital aniridia. A novel heterozygous frameshift mutation (c.391_398dupATACCAAG, p.Ser133Argfs*8) in exon 7 of the *PAX6* gene was identified in all affected individuals in the family. This study demonstrates that this frameshift mutation of the *PAX6* gene might be the causative genetic defect of congenital aniridia in this family. This mutation is predicted to cause the premature truncation of the PAX6 protein, leading to the functional haploinsufficiency of PAX6, which may be the major molecular mechanism underlying the aniridia phenotype. To the best of our knowledge, this is the first report of a novel pathogenic *PAX6* gene variant c.391_398dupATACCAAG(p.Ser133Argfs*8) identified in a Chinese family with congenital aniridia.

Keywords: aniridia; *PAX6* gene; targeted gene capture sequencing; frameshift; autosomal recessive inheritance

Citation: Wang, C.; Yang, W.; Li, X.; Zhou, C.; Liu, J.; Jin, L.; Jiang, Q.; Wang, Y. A Novel *PAX6* Frameshift Mutation Identified in a Large Chinese Family with Congenital Aniridia. *J. Pers. Med.* **2023**, *13*, 442. https://doi.org/10.3390/jpm13030442

Academic Editors: Kai Jin and Chun Zhang

Received: 11 January 2023
Revised: 25 February 2023
Accepted: 26 February 2023
Published: 28 February 2023

1. Introduction

Congenital aniridia (MIM 106210) is a rare panocular malformation with an incidence ranging from 1:64,000 to 1:100,000. It is characterized by either an absence or hypoplasia of the iris in both eyes [1]. It usually occurs with other ocular abnormalities such as cataracts, aniridia-related keratopathy, glaucoma, nystagmus, foveal hypoplasia, and obvious visual impairment. Congenital aniridia manifests in different forms, most of which are transmitted in an autosomal-dominant manner with a high degree of penetrance. It can also be sporadic, and as part of several syndromes including WAGR and WAGRO syndromes, as well as other syndromes with an intellectual impairment [2]. Studies have showed that about two-thirds of aniridia cases are familial, and the remaining one-third are sporadic [3]. The majority of congenital aniridia and other ocular disorders such as Peters anomaly occur due to different mutations found in or around the transcription factor *PAX6* gene (paired box 6, MIM 607108). The mutations reported in this gene are scattered throughout the complete coding sequence of the gene or in the regulatory regions. The mutations in the *PAX6* gene cause ocular abnormalities including aniridia in both vertebrate and invertebrate animal species. Studies have reported that the majority of *PAX6* mutations are heterozygous, resulting in the loss of one allele causing *PAX6* haploinsufficiency [4].

The *PAX6* gene is highly conserved throughout biological functions across diverse species, implicating its key role in embryonal ocular differentiation. It encodes a transcription factor, which is a 2.7 kb mRNA encoding a 422-amino-acid protein. It contains two DNA-binding domains: the paired domain (PD) and the homeodomain (HD). They are isolated by a linker segment (LNK), followed by a C-terminal region, rich in proline, serine, and threonine (PST) [5–7], which is a transactivation domain.

Numerous researchers have proven that the PAX6 protein is crucial for the normal development and maintenance of the eye, central nervous system, and many other elements [8–11]. Notably, *PAX6* is identified as the master gene controlling eye development. It is expressed in most ocular structures and plays key roles in lens induction, epithelial tissue morphogenesis, and neuronal specification or differentiation [12]. Mutations in the *PAX6* gene cause a series of ocular diseases, such as nystagmus, cataracts, and aniridia [13]. In recent years, many studies have focused on the varied clinical manifestation and allelic heterogeneity of *PAX6*-associated aniridia. In this study, a clinical and genetic evaluation of a four-generation Chinese family with congenital aniridia was carried out. A novel heterozygous frameshift mutation of the *PAX6* gene was identified. The molecular understanding of the predicted impact based on existing research and prediction algorithms was clarified. Moreover, the available clinical features of *PAX6*-associated aniridia in this study were investigated. To the best of our knowledge, this is the first reported association of the *PAX6* gene variant c.391_398dupATACCAAG, p.Ser133Argfs*8 with congenital aniridia.

2. Materials and Methods

2.1. Human Subjects

A four-consecutive-generation Han Chinese pedigree (Figure 1) with congenital aniridia was recruited from The Affiliated Eye Hospital of Nanjing Medical University for the study. This family contained 29 individuals including 13 patients and 16 unaffected individuals. All procedures performed in studies involving human participants were in accordance with the ethical standards of the institutional and/or national research committee and with the 1964 Helsinki Declaration and its later amendments or comparable ethical standards. The study was approved by the Medical Ethics Committee of Eye Hospital, Nanjing Medical University (No. 2019004). Informed written consent was obtained from all participants prior to inclusion in the study.

2.2. Clinical Evaluation

All members recruited in this study underwent thorough ophthalmic examinations, including uncorrected and best-corrected visual acuity (BCVA), slit-lamp biomicroscopy of the anterior segment, eye position, eyeball movement, fundus examination after dilation, intraocular pressure (IOP) measurement, and optical coherence tomography.

2.3. Genomic DNA Extraction and DNA Library Preparation

After informed consent, blood samples were collected from all unrelated aniridia patients and most unaffected family members for DNA extraction and genomic analysis. The genomic DNA of all individuals was extracted from 2 mL of peripheral venous blood using a Blood Genomic DNA Extraction Kit (CoWin Bioscience, Beijing, China) according to the manufacturer's instructions. DNA integrity was evaluated via 1% agarose gel electrophoresis. Targeted gene enrichment and sequencing were performed on the proband IV8. Genomic DNA was fragmented to an average size of 180 bp with sonication. Paired-end sequencing library preparation, comprising end repair, adapter ligation, and PCR enrichment, were carried out as recommended by Illumina protocols using DNA sample prep reagent set 1 (New England Biolabs (Beijing) LTD., Beijing, China).

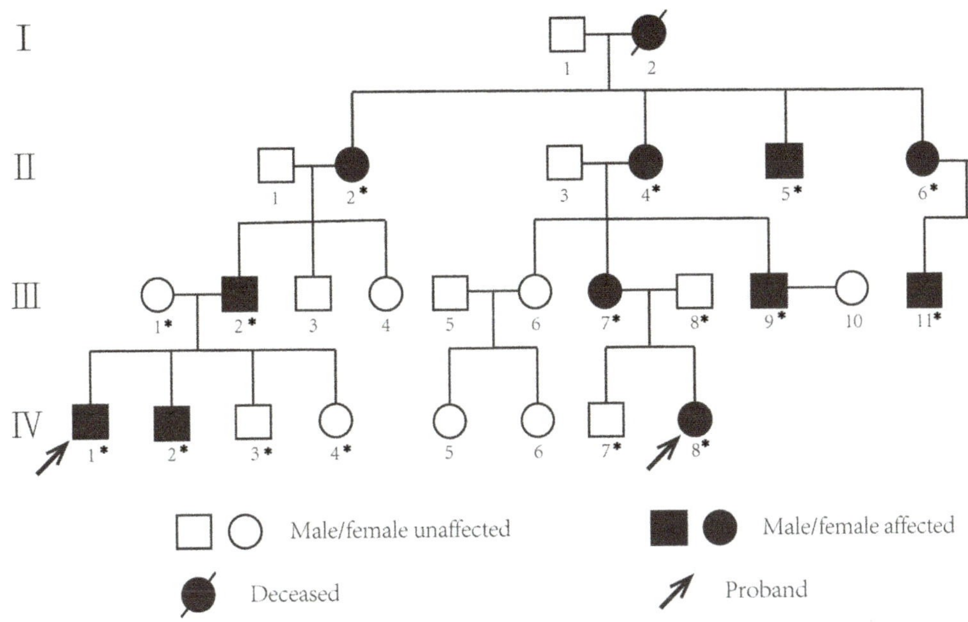

Figure 1. Pedigree of a Chinese family with congenital aniridia. Filled squares and circles denote affected males and females, respectively. Normal individuals are shown as empty symbols. The proband is indicated by an arrow. DNA samples used for sanger sequencing are marked with an asterisk.

2.4. Targeted Gene Enrichment and Sequencing

Targeted next-generation sequencing (NGS) was carried out with DNA probes designed to tile along the exon regions of 815 known pathogenic genes of hereditary ophthalmic disorders (Table S1), and the amplified DNA was captured using a GenCap capture kit (MyGenostics, Beijing, China) depending on the manufacturer's instructions. The PCR product was purified by SPRI beads (Beckman Instruments, Brea, CA, USA) according to the manufacturer's protocol. The enrichment libraries were sequenced on an Illumina HiSeq X ten sequencer (Illumina, San Diego, CA, USA) for 150 bp paired reads. Mutations were called after sequencing using BWA (http://bio-bwa.sourceforge.net/, accessed on 25 February 2023) and GATK (https://gatk.broadinstitute.org/hc/en-us, accessed on 25 February 2023) and annotated using ANNOVAR (http://annovar.openbioinformatics.org/en/latest/, accessed on 25 February 2023). The filtering process included all coding variants with an MAF < 5% and excluded synonymous and in-frame insertion/deletion variants. The identified mutation was named according to the nomenclature established by the Human Genomic Variation Society (HGVS). Candidate genes and variants were analyzed in combination with the patients' phenotypes and public variant databases. Pathogenic genes and genetic variations with known, definitive genetic associations with aniridia were paid more attention, including *PAX6*, *ABCB6*, *FOXC1*, *PITX2*, *FOXD3*, and *CYP1B1*.

2.5. Sanger Sequencing

Direct Sanger sequencing was performed to determine the co-segregation of identified variants with the clinical phenotype in all affected family members and some normal members. The primer flanking region on exon 7 of the *PAX6* gene that covers the mutation Primers (5′–TGAAAGTATCATCATATTTGTAG–3′ (F) and 5′–AGGAGAGAGCATTGGGCTTA–3′ (R)) were designed using Primer Premier 5 and synthesized by BGI (Guangzhou, China). Polymerase chain reaction (PCR) was performed using a MyCycler thermal cycler

(Bio-Rad, Hercules, CA, USA) in a 25 μL reaction system, which contained 0.1 μg of genomic DNA, 40 μmol/L forward and reverse primers, 3 mmol/L magnesiumchloride, and 2× Taq Master Mix (SinoBio, Shanghai, China). The PCR conditions used were as follows: 4 min at 95 °C for initial denaturation, 35 cycles of denaturation at 95 °C for 10 s for melting, annealing temperature of 54 °C lasting for 30 s, 30 s at 72 °C for extension and a final additional extension step of 5 min at 72 °C. Before sequencing, 1% agarose gel electrophoresis was used to purify the target PCR fragments using the QIAquick Gel Extraction Kit (QIAGEN, Shanghai, China). Sanger sequencing was performed on a 3130XL sequencer and analyzed on an ABI 3130 Genetic Analyzer (Applied Biosystems, Thermo Fisher Scientific, Waltham, MA, USA). Sequence data were compared in a pairwise manner with the related human genome database (Assembly GRCh37/hg19).

2.6. Variant Analyses

To analyze the evolutionary conservation of the mutant region, the sequences of *PAX6* orthologs in different vertebrate species were retrieved from the NCBI Reference Sequence database. A multiple alignment of homologous sequences from eight species was conducted using ClustalW2 (http://www.ebi.ac.uk/Tools/msa/clustalw2/, accessed on 25 February 2023). ACMG Guidelines were used through various algorithms for prediction of the impact of the variant on protein structure and the prediction of pathogenicity. Additionally, protein three-dimensional structures of full-length and mutated *PAX6* were evaluated with the Swiss-Model program (https://swissmodel.expasy.org/interactive, accessed on 25 February 2023).

3. Results

3.1. Clinical Features of the Family with Congenital Aniridia

The four-generation Chinese family enrolled in this study consisted of 29 individuals (Figure 1) with 13 patients diagnosed as congenital aniridia (I2 died). The probands IV1 and IV8 came to the hospital for treatment much earlier. Among all thirteen patients, seven (53.8%) were female, while the remaining six (46.2%) were male, with their ages varying from 3 to 69. All the affected members exhibited almost similar ocular symptoms, including complete absence of the irises, horizontal tremor, foveal hypoplasia, and uncorrected visual impairment in both eyes. Interestingly, peripheral corneal edema and opacification was observed in seven relatively older patients (53.8%), while lens opacity was also present in seven of thirteen patients (53.8%), indicating a positive correlation with age. In this respect, patient III2 deserved attention due to the experience of bilateral cataract surgery. Four of thirteen affected individuals (30.8%) suffered from strabismus, two (III2, III9) of thirteen patients (15.4%) suffered from exotropia, and the remaining two (II2, IV8) of thirteen patients (15.4%) suffered from esotropia. Except for proband IV1 who complained of ptosis, no other ocular or systemic abnormalities were detected. Ophthalmic manifestations of all patients and representative examination results are shown in Figure 2 and Table 1.

3.2. Molecular Analysis

NGS was implemented for proband IV8. Detailed information about the sequencing and alignment quality of NGS data is provided in Table S2. Following NGS and the data analysis, a heterozygous frameshift mutation of the *PAX6* gene (NM_001604) was detected in proband IV8. *PAX6* was the most likely pathogenic gene in this study, which is further elaborated on in the discussion. This mutation (c.391_398dupATACCAAG, p.Ser133Argfs*8) was neither present in the databases of 1000 genome, ESP6500, dbSNP, EXAC, and HGMD, nor reported previously. To verify the identified gene defects, PCR and Sanger sequencing were applied to DNA samples, including 12 affected individuals and 5 unaffected family members who were available (Figure S1). The results manifested that all individuals with congenital aniridia of the pedigree harbored this heterozygous mutation. Diametrically, unaffected family members did not carry the variant (Figure 3). In brief, this mutation was co-segregated with the disease phenotype with complete penetrance.

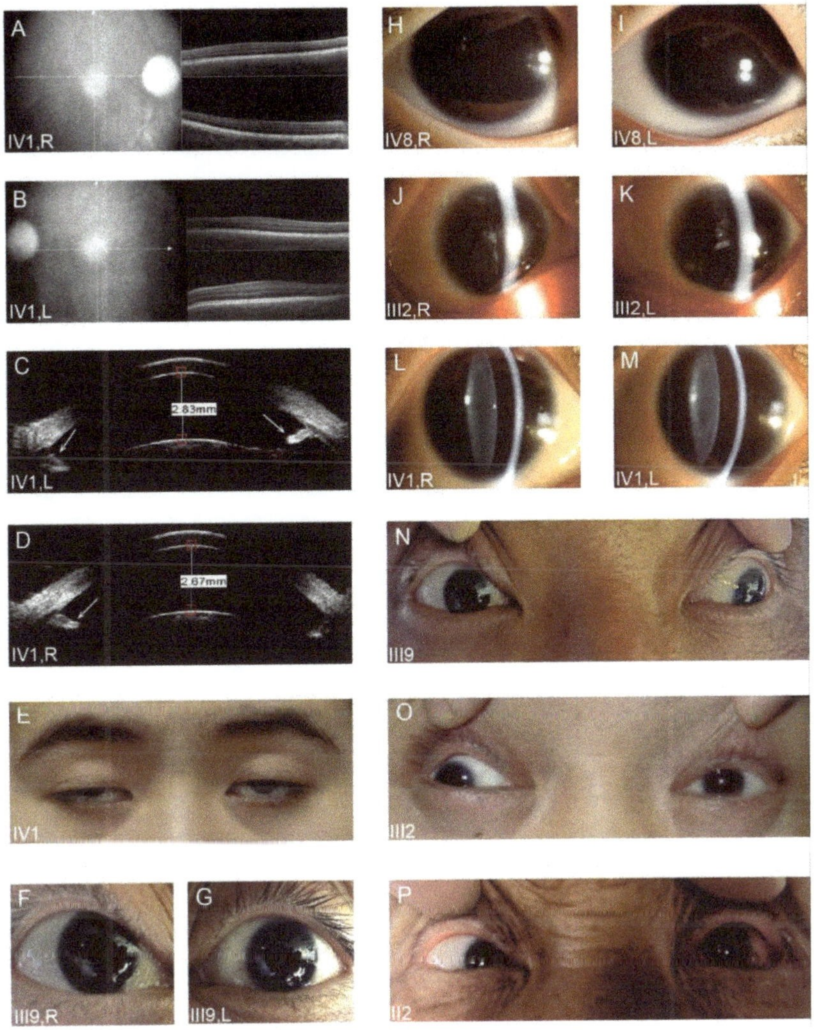

Figure 2. Representative photos of partial cases. (**A**,**B**) Optical coherence tomography images from the proband (IV1) demonstrated foveal hypoplasia in both the right eye (**A**) and the left eye (**B**). (**C**,**D**) Ultrasound biomicroscope photos displayed the iris remnants (the arrow) in the anterior chamber of the proband (IV1) in both eyes. (**E**) Ptosis was present in the proband (IV1). (**F**,**G**) Photos revealed total iris hypoplasia in both eyes of patient III9. (**H**,**I**) Anterior segment photographs indicated that both eyes of the proband IV8 exhibited complete iris absence. (**J**,**K**) The eyes of patient III2 were found with peripheral corneal edema and opacity, total iris hypoplasia, and aphakia by anterior segment photography. (**L**,**M**) Bilateral aniridia and cataract were observed in the proband (IV1). (**N**,**O**,**P**) Eye position photographs manifested that patient III9 (**N**) and patient III2 (**O**) suffered from exotropia, while patient II2 (**P**) developed esotropia.

Table 1. Clinical details of patients of the recruited family.

Pedigree Number	Gender	Age (Years)	BCVA (OD/OS)	IOP (mmHg) (OD/OS)	Aniridia	KP	Cataract	Macular Foveal Reflect	Nystagmus	Strabismus
II2	F	69	CF (20 cm)/0.12	21/19	Total	Corneal edema and opacity	+	–	+	Esotropia
II4	F	63	0.15/0.04	18/22	Total	Corneal edema and opacity	+	–	+	–
II5	M	59	0.02/CF (30 cm)	18/16	Total	Corneal edema and opacity	+	–	+	–
II6	F	50	0.06/CF (30 cm)	17/19	Total	Corneal edema and opacity	+	–	+	–
III2	M	46	0.01/CF (20 cm)	15/16	Total	Corneal edema and opacity	Aphakia	–	+	Exotropia
III7	F	34	0.12/0.1	20/21	Total	Corneal edema and opacity	+	–	+	–
III9	M	30	0.1/0.2	19/18	Total	Corneal edema and opacity	–	–	+	Exotropia
III11	M	24	0.3/0.3	17/20	Total	–	+	–	+	–
III12	F	20	0.06/0.1	18/19	Total	–	–	–	+	–
IV1	M	19	0.2/0.2	20/18	Total	–	+	–	+	–
IV2	M	3	0.1/0.3	16/17	Total	–	–	–	+	–
IV8	F	6	0.1-/0.1	19/19	Total	–	–	–	+	Esotropia

Abbreviations: M: male; F: female; BCVA: best-corrected visual acuity; CF: count fingers; OD: oculus dexter; OS: oculus sinister.

The *PAX6* gene variant (c.391_398dupATACCAAG, p.Ser133Argfs*8) was located in exon 7. This 8-bp duplication converts serine to arginine at amino-acid position 133, followed by another seven erroneous residues, and was predicted to create a truncated protein with 125 amino acids (Figure 4B) in comparison with a full-length wildtype protein of *PAX6* with 436 amino acids (Figure 4A). According to ACMG/AMP Guidelines for genomic variant classification, this variation was assessed for "pathogenic" with evidence of pathogenicity: PVS1, PM2, PP1, and PP4 (Table 2).

It was demonstrated that the serine at position 133 of PAX6 was highly conserved during evolution using ClustalW2 with multiple alignments of orthologs from eight different species: rabbit, tropical clawed frog, chicken, house mouse, dog, cattle, human, and Norway rat (Figure 4B). Bioinformatics analysis showed that the duplication of ATACCAAG at position c.391_398 may disrupt the open reading frames of *PAX6*, possibly retaining most of the paired domain of PAX6 but lacking the remaining domains, including the linker segment, the homeodomain, and the PST domain. Like other *PAX6* frameshift variants reported, this very likely causes haploinsufficiency due to nonsense-mediated decay (NMD). Even if the mutant transcript escapes NMD, the protein is expected to be nonfunctional. Swiss-Model predicted the 3D structure of PAX6 from the N terminal. The results indicated that mutated PAX6 even loses the α-helix of the paired domain (Figure 5), which may not be expected to be produced. The truncated protein might be unable to perform its substantial biological functions in ocular and neurologic development. Taken together, this variant of *PAX6* is a novel mutation which was most likely responsible for autosomal dominant congenital aniridia in this study.

Table 2. Summary of the *PAX6* gene and its variant.

Gene	Position	Transcript	Exon	Change of Nucleotide	Predicted Change of Amino Acid	Domain	Variant Type	Status	ACMG/AMP Variant Classification
PAX6	chr11:31823109 *	NM_001604	7	c.391_398dupATACCAAG	p.Ser133Argfs*8	PD	Frameshift	Het	Pathogenic #

* Assembly GRCh37/hg19. # Evidence of pathogenicity: PVS1 + PM2 + PP1 + PP4. Abbreviations: Het, heterozygous; PD: paired domain.

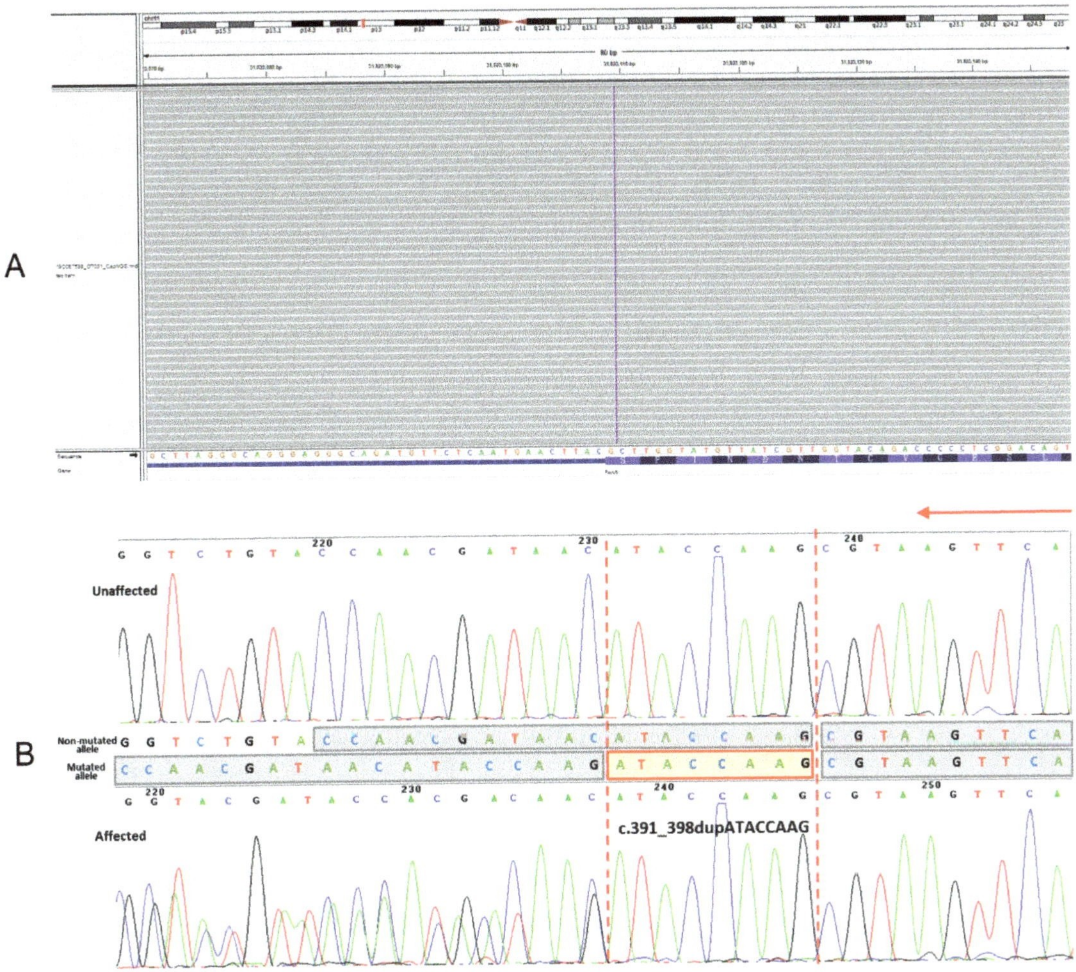

Figure 3. Sequencing results for the variant c.391_398dupATACCAAG of the *PAX6* gene. (**A**) Integrative genomics viewer visualization of whole-exome sequencing showing a novel heterozygous variant in the *PAX6* gene in the proband (IV8). (**B**) Sanger sequencing results of the *PAX6* gene confirmed the mutant allele with ATACCAAG duplicated at the position indicating by two red dotted line, in the affected individuals represented in the lower panel versus the normal individuals in the upper panel. Sequencing direction is indicated by an red arrow.

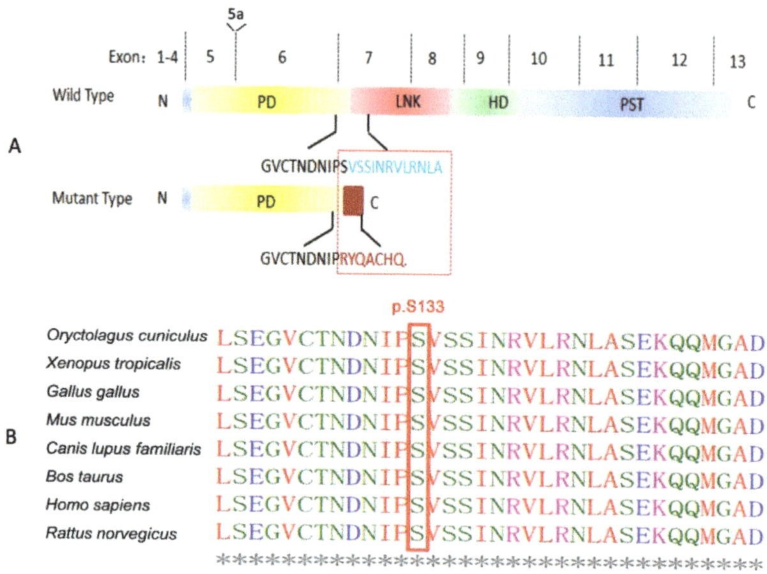

Figure 4. Schematic of predicted mutant PAX6 protein and bioinformatics analysis following ClustalW alignment. (**A**) Schematic of mutant PAX6 protein (lower panel) as predicted in this study compared with the wildtype PAX6 protein (upper panel). N, N terminus; PD, paired domain; LNK, linker domain; HD, homeodomain; PST, proline, serine, and threonine-rich domain; C, C terminus. Due to the frameshift duplication, the peptide in blue encoded by exon 7 of the wildtype is replaced by the peptide in red in the mutant in the box. (**B**) The *PAX6* mutation c.391_398dupATACCAAG involves a highly conserved residue. The serine at position 133 is highly conserved for PAX6, as demonstrated by an analysis of orthologs from eight different species: rabbit, tropical clawed frog, chicken, house mouse, dog, cattle, human, and Norway rat.

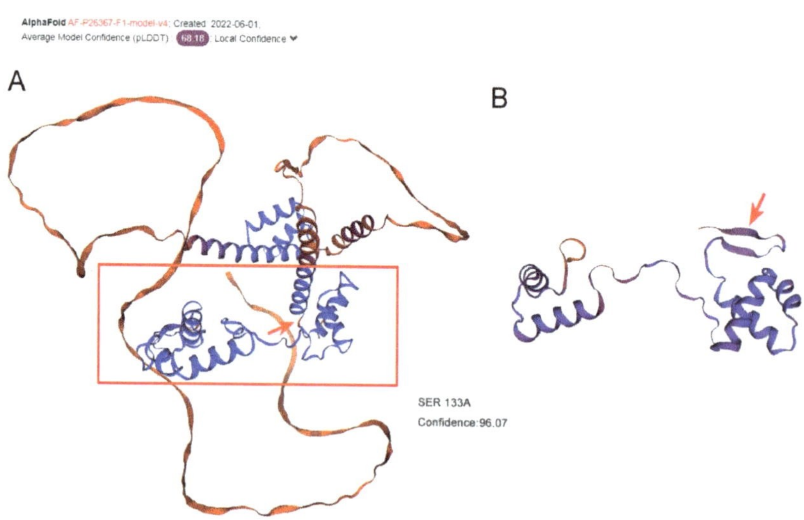

Figure 5. Three-dimensional structure prediction of wildtype PAX6 and mutated PAX6 protein. (**A**) Wildtype PAX6 structure. (**B**) Mutated PAX6 structure. The red arrow indicates the mutated position S133.

4. Discussion

The *PAX6* gene, considered a causative gene for congenital aniridia since 1991 [6], is located at chromosome 11p13 in the assembly GRCh37/hg19, consists of 14 exons and 13 introns, and encodes 3 isoforms of transcripts determined by alternative splicing, including 1 isoform with an alternative exon between exon 5 and 6, called exon 5a [14]. The translation initiation codon is in exon 4, and the termination codon is in exon 14, with the first 3 being noncoding (Figure 5A). The alternative exonic inclusion of exon 5a generates a larger protein isoform PAX6-5a of 436 amino acids (NM_001604). It is highly conserved throughout biological evolution across different species, encoding a transcription factor which can initiate and regulate the transcription of downstream genes during embryogenesis via attaching to special areas of DNA [15]. PAX6 is expressed in almost all ocular structures including the iris, macula, optic nerve head, lens, and cornea [2,7], playing a key role in early eye development. PAX6 regulates the tissue-specific expression of different molecules, hormones, and structural proteins, and the transcription of target genes can only be initiated when the expression of PAX6 reaches a certain dose [16]. Mutations in the *PAX6* gene cause anterior segment malformations including aniridia, accompanied by a range of ocular phenotypes such as keratitis, cataract, glaucoma, nystagmus, foveal hypoplasia, and optic nerve disorders.

In this study, a novel heterozygous frameshift mutation of the *PAX6* gene (c.391_398dup ATACCAAG, p.Ser133Argfs*8) was identified in a Chinese family. The genomic defects were present in all affected members but absent in unaffected family members, co-segregating with congenital aniridia, which is consistent with the previously reported pedigree. A small duplication of an ATACCAAG sequence at nucleotide position 391 of PAX6 was predicted to cause the replacement of a negatively charged serine by a positively charged arginine and generating or forming a premature stop signal eight codons downstream in exon 7. This altered the original open reading frame, which was expected to truncate PAX6 protein within the linker region. The resulting polypeptide then possibly retained the paired domain but lacked the homeodomain, the PST domain, and almost the entire linker segment. To our knowledge, outside of the homeodomain which combines with DNA directly, the PST domain is indispensable by acting as a strong activator, according to a single report which compared the transcriptional activation between wildtype and mutant PAX6 PST domains [7]. Researchers studied the attachment of wildtype or mutant PAX6 protein (TGA306 or TGA353) to the DNA-binding site of yeast GAL4, and then combined them with a plasmid containing the chloramphenicol acetyltransferase (CAT) gene. It was revealed that one mutant fusion protein (TGA353) stimulated CAT expression at only 5–10% of the wildtype level, whereas the other had no detectable CAT activity. Without testing, the novel mutation we described in this study truncated the PAX6 protein further upstream than what was examined in the mentioned article. Hence, it is highly possible that it eliminated the transcription activity. Although the DNA interaction is unlikely to be totally abolished as the paired domains are still there for DNA binding, we believe that the mutation has a non-negligible, negative affect, even deteriorating the function of remaining paired domains. Swiss-Model, sufficient for three-dimensional structure prediction, gave evidence which supports our conjecture [17–20]. It showed an apparent α-helix deletion (Figure 4), which contributes to the malformed PAX6 protein space structure and may perturb the affinity and specificity of DNA interaction, resulting in a decrease in protein function. On a gross level, the findings elucidated above may partially explain the molecular mechanisms of congenital aniridia.

Previous studies showed a wide spectrum of clinical manifestations accompanying aniridia, such as cataract, keratopathy, glaucoma, nystagmus, foveal hypoplasia, and low vision acuity [2,21]. Noticeably, phenotypes are severe when crossing onto an insertion/duplication mutation background [22]. Consistent with this, all mutation carriers in the family we recruited developed a complete loss of the iris, foveal hypoplasia, horizontal tremor, and vision impairment. A particularly compelling finding is that patients with the same mutation can exhibit various aniridia phenotypes, even in the same family. Available data of genotype and phenotype allowed for an exhaustive investigation in the pedigree we observed. Some associated diseases occurred in some, but not all individuals. Only four patients exhibited strabismus, while another one was diagnosed with ptosis. Among the members who suffered from corneal and/or lens opacity, the damage deteriorated with age. Regarding this phenomenon, we inferred that it may have derived from the haploinsufficiency of PAX6. Although many of these clinical features are present at birth, some can develop and/or progress later in life [11]. In addition to its activity in the embryo, PAX6 is maintained in specific cell types of the adult eye, including the corneal limbus, the iris, the pigmented ciliary body, the lens epithelium, and the Muller glia. This demonstrates that PAX6 activity may be implicated in adult self-renewal and regeneration of ocular structures, considering the functions of these cells [12]. Another alternative interpretation would be the NMD process. This pathway degrades some transcripts, bearing a premature translational termination codon, which aggravates or counteracts the effects of disease mutations [23]. These findings may partly reflect genetic heterogeneity; however, fully understanding the molecular mechanism remains a formidable challenge.

Until now, 550 mutations of the *PAX6* gene have been featured in the public version of the HGMD (http://www.hgmd.cf.ac.uk/ac/gene.php?gene=PAX6, accessed on 25 February 2023). These mutations are mainly devoted to aniridia, Peters abnormalities, foveal hypoplasia, nystagmus, cataracts, optic nerve dysplasia, and other eye diseases [13]. Roughly 30.0% are missense and nonsense mutations, while 11.6% are splicing site mutations. Small fragment deletions and insertions account for 23.6% and 10.5%, respectively. The remaining 20.2% of mutations are regulatory, gross duplication, complex rearrangements and other rare mutation types. Mutation types including nonsense and frameshift (insertions, duplication or deletions) will introduce a PTC and a consequent termination of translation, which are most commonly found in *PAX6*. In the present study, duplication mutation c.391_398dupATACCAAG of the *PAX6* gene results in a replacement of the subsequent amino-acid residues from position p.S133 with a peptide of eight erroneous amino-acid residues, including a PTC at the end. Singh and his colleagues demonstrated a dominant-negative mechanism using transient transfection assays with a variety of mutant PAX6 proteins featuring the C terminus half-truncated, co-expressed with wildtype PAX6 protein. All these mutant proteins lose most of the transactivation domain (PST), thereby acting as a repressor with no transactivation activity, but still maintaining DNA-binding domains (PD and HD) [24].

5. Conclusions

In summary, we analyzed the ocular phenotypes of 13 aniridia patients and identified a novel *PAX6* frameshift mutation as the causative gene defect in a four-generation Chinese family. This is a novel pathogenic mutation related to aniridia. Although the definite mechanism underlying how this variant in exon 7 of the *PAX6* gene triggers congenital aniridia is not yet clear, our study contributes additional information for future research. It expands the mutation spectrum of *PAX6*-related congenital aniridia, which is beneficial for prenatal diagnosis, genetic counseling, and gene therapy for familial cases in the near future. In addition, the molecular mechanism of genotype–phenotype correlations needs to be further investigated.

Supplementary Materials: The following supporting information can be downloaded at: https://www.mdpi.com/article/10.3390/jpm13030442/s1, Table S1. Known pathogenic gene list of hereditary ophthalmic disorders; Table S2. Detail information about NGS data of proband IV8. Figure S1. Sanger sequencing results of *PAX6* gene on DNA samples from affected individuals and most family members who were available.

Author Contributions: Conceptualization, W.Y., Q.J. and Y.W.; formal analysis, C.W., W.Y. and Y.W.; investigation, C.W., X.L., C.Z., J.L. and L.J.; writing—original draft, C.W.; writing—review and editing, Q.J. and Y.W. All authors have read and agreed to the published version of the manuscript.

Funding: This work was supported by the National Natural Science Foundation of China (81800858), the Science and Technology Innovation Committee of Shenzhen (Grant no. JCYJ20210324125614039), the Scientific Research Project of the Chinese Medicine Education Association (2022KTM028), the Shenzhen Fund for Guangdong Provincial High-level Clinical Key Specialties (SZGSP014), and the Sanming Project of Medicine in Shenzhen (SZSM202011015).

Institutional Review Board Statement: The study was conducted in accordance with the Declaration of Helsinki and approved by the Medical Ethics Committee of Eye Hospital, Nanjing Medical University (No.2019004).

Informed Consent Statement: Informed consent was obtained from all subjects involved in the study.

Data Availability Statement: The data presented in this study are available on request from the corresponding author.

Conflicts of Interest: The authors declare no conflict of interest.

References

1. Ugalahi, M.O.; Ibukun, F.A.; Olusanya, B.A.; Baiyeroju, A.M. Congenital aniridia: Clinical profile of children seen at the University College Hospital, Ibadan, South-West Nigeria. *Ther. Adv. Ophthalmol.* **2021**, *13*, 25158414211019513. [CrossRef]
2. Lagali, N.; Wowra, B.; Fries, F.N.; Latta, L.; Moslemani, K.; Utheim, T.P.; Wylegala, E.; Seitz, B.; Käsmann-Kellner, B. Early phenotypic features of aniridia-associated keratopathy and association with PAX6 coding mutations. *Ocul. Surf.* **2019**, *18*, 130–140. [CrossRef]
3. Landsend, E.C.S.; Pedersen, H.R.; Utheim, A.; Rueegg, C.S.; Baraas, R.C.; Lagali, N.; Bragadóttir, R.; Moe, M.C.; Utheim, T.P. Characteristics and Utility of Fundus Autofluorescence in Congenital Aniridia Using Scanning Laser Ophthalmoscopy. *Investig. Opthalmology Vis. Sci.* **2019**, *60*, 4120–4128. [CrossRef]
4. Pedersen, H.R.; Baraas, R.C.; Landsend, E.C.S.; Utheim, A.; Utheim, T.P.; Gilson, S.J.; Neitz, M. *PAX6* Genotypic and Retinal Phenotypic Characterization in Congenital Aniridia. *Investig. Opthalmology Vis. Sci.* **2020**, *61*, 14. [CrossRef]
5. Glaser, T.; Walton, D.S.; Maas, R.L. Genomic structure, evolutionary conservation and aniridia mutations in the human PAX6 gene. *Nat. Genet.* **1992**, *2*, 232–239. [CrossRef]
6. Ton, C.C.; Hirvonen, H.; Miwa, H.; Weil, M.M.; Monaghan, P.; Jordan, T.; van Heyningen, V.; Hastie, N.D.; Meijers-Heijboer, H.; Drechsler, M.; et al. Positional cloning and characterization of a paired box- and homeobox-containing gene from the aniridia region. *Cell* **1991**, *67*, 1059–1074. [CrossRef]
7. Glaser, T.; Jepeal, L.; Edwards, J.G.; Young, S.R.; Favor, J.; Maas, R.L. PAX6 gene dosage effect in a family with congenital cataracts, aniridia, anophthalmia and central nervous system defects. *Nat. Genet.* **1994**, *7*, 463–471. [CrossRef]
8. Latta, L.; Ludwig, N.; Krammes, L.; Stachon, T.; Fries, F.; Mukwaya, A.; Szentmáry, N.; Seitz, B.; Wowra, B.; Kahraman, M.; et al. Abnormal neovascular and proliferative conjunctival phenotype in limbal stem cell deficiency is associated with altered microRNA and gene expression modulated by PAX6 mutational status in congenital aniridia. *Ocul. Surf.* **2021**, *19*, 115–127. [CrossRef]
9. Xiao, Y.; Liu, X.; Yang, C.; Liu, L.; Guo, X.; Wang, Q.; Gong, B. A Novel *PAX6* Heterozygous Mutation Found in a Chinese Family with Congenital Aniridia. *Genet. Test. Mol. Biomarkers* **2019**, *23*, 495–500. [CrossRef]
10. Thakurela, S.; Tiwari, N.; Schick, S.; Garding, A.; Ivanek, R.; Berninger, B.; Tiwari, V.K. Mapping gene regulatory circuitry of Pax6 during neurogenesis. *Cell Discov.* **2016**, *2*, 15045. [CrossRef]
11. Rabiee, B.; Anwar, K.N.; Shen, X.; Putra, I.; Liu, M.; Jung, R.; Afsharkhamseh, N.; Rosenblatt, M.I.; Fishman, G.A.; Liu, X.; et al. Gene dosage manipulation alleviates manifestations of hereditary *PAX6* haploinsufficiency in mice. *Sci. Transl. Med.* **2020**, *12*, eaaz4894. [CrossRef] [PubMed]
12. Shaham, O.; Menuchin, Y.; Farhy, C.; Ashery-Padan, R. Pax6: A multi-level regulator of ocular development. *Prog. Retin. Eye Res.* **2012**, *31*, 351–376. [CrossRef] [PubMed]
13. Hingorani, M.; Hanson, I.; van Heyningen, V. Aniridia. *Eur. J. Hum. Genet. EJHG.* **2012**, *20*, 1011–1017. [CrossRef] [PubMed]
14. Chalepakis, G.; Stoykova, A.; Wijnholds, J.; Tremblay, P.; Gruss, P. Pax: Gene regulators in the developing nervous system. *J. Neurobiol.* **1993**, *24*, 1367–1384. [CrossRef]
15. Plaisancié, J.; Tarilonte, M.; Ramos, P.; Jeanton-Scaramouche, C.; Gaston, V.; Dollfus, H.; Aguilera, D.; Kaplan, J.; Fares-Taie, L.; Blanco-Kelly, F.; et al. Implication of non-coding PAX6 mutations in aniridia. *Hum. Genet.* **2018**, *137*, 831–846. [CrossRef]
16. Kokotas, H.; Petersen, M.B. Clinical and molecular aspects of aniridia. *Clin. Genet.* **2010**, *77*, 409–420. [CrossRef]
17. Biasini, M.; Bienert, S.; Waterhouse, A.; Arnold, K.; Studer, G.; Schmidt, T.; Kiefer, F.; Cassarino, T.G.; Bertoni, M.; Bordoli, L.; et al. SWISS-MODEL: Modelling protein tertiary and quaternary structure using evolutionary information. *Nucleic Acids Res.* **2014**, *42*, W252–W258. [CrossRef]
18. Kiefer, F.; Arnold, K.; Künzli, M.; Bordoli, L.; Schwede, T. The SWISS-MODEL Repository and associated resources. *Nucleic Acids Res.* **2009**, *37*, D387–D392. [CrossRef]
19. Arnold, K.; Bordoli, L.; Kopp, J.; Schwede, T. The SWISS-MODEL workspace: A web-based environment for protein structure homology modelling. *Bioinformatics* **2006**, *22*, 195–201. [CrossRef]

20. Guex, N.; Peitsch, M.C.; Schwede, T. Automated comparative protein structure modeling with SWISS-MODEL and Swiss-PdbViewer: A historical perspective. *Electrophoresis* **2009**, *30* (Suppl. S1), S162–S173. [CrossRef]
21. Filatova, A.Y.; Vasilyeva, T.A.; Marakhonov, A.V.; Sukhanova, N.V.; Voskresenskaya, A.A.; Zinchenko, R.A.; Skoblov, M.Y. Upstream ORF frameshift variants in the PAX6 5′UTR cause congenital aniridia. *Hum. Mutat.* **2021**, *42*, 1053–1065. [CrossRef] [PubMed]
22. Villarroel, C.E.; Villanueva-Mendoza, C.; Orozco, L.; Alcántara-Ortigoza, M.A.; Jiménez, D.F.; Ordaz, J.C.; Angel, A.G.-D. Molecular analysis of the PAX6 gene in Mexican patients with congenital aniridia: Report of four novel mutations. *Mol. Vis.* **2008**, *14*, 1650–1658. [PubMed]
23. Supek, F.; Lehner, B.; Lindeboom, R.G.H. To NMD or Not To NMD: Nonsense-Mediated mRNA Decay in Cancer and Other Genetic Diseases. *Trends Genet. TIG* **2021**, *37*, 657–668. [CrossRef] [PubMed]
24. Singh, S.; Tang, H.K.; Lee, J.-Y.; Saunders, G.F. Truncation Mutations in the Transactivation Region of PAX6 Result in Dominant-Negative Mutants. *J. Biol. Chem.* **1998**, *273*, 21531–21541. [CrossRef] [PubMed]

Journal of
Personalized
Medicine

MDPI

Article

MAC-ResNet: Knowledge Distillation Based Lightweight Multiscale-Attention-Crop-ResNet for Eyelid Tumors Detection and Classification

Xingru Huang [1,2], Chunlei Yao [3], Feng Xu [4], Lingxiao Chen [4], Huaqiong Wang [1], Xiaodiao Chen [1,4], Juan Ye [3] and Yaqi Wang [1,*]

1 College of Media Engineering, Communication University of Zhejiang, Hangzhou 310042, China; xingru.huang@qmul.ac.uk (X.H.); wanghuaqiong@cuz.edu.cn (H.W.); xiaodiao@hdu.edu.cn (X.C.)
2 School of Electronic Engineering and Computer Science, Queen Mary University of London, Mile End Road, London E1 4NS, UK
3 Department of Ophthalmology, The Second Affiliated Hospital of Zhejiang University School of Medicine, Hangzhou 310009, China; chunleiyao@zju.edu.cn (C.Y.); yejuan@zju.edu.cn (J.Y.)
4 School of Computer Science and Technology, Hangzhou Dianzi University, Hangzhou 310005, China; 222050141@hdu.edu.cn (F.X.); lingxiao@hdu.edu.cn (L.C.)
* Correspondence: wangyaqi@cuz.edu.cn

Abstract: Eyelid tumors are tumors that occur in the eye and its appendages, affecting vision and appearance, causing blindness and disability, and some having a high lethality rate. Pathological images of eyelid tumors are characterized by large pixels, multiple scales, and similar features. Solving the problem of difficult and time-consuming fine-grained classification of pathological images is important to improve the efficiency and quality of pathological diagnosis. The morphology of Basal Cell Carcinoma (BCC), Meibomian Gland Carcinoma (MGC), and Cutaneous Melanoma (CM) in eyelid tumors are very similar, and it is easy to be misdiagnosed among each category. In addition, the diseased area, which is decisive for the diagnosis of the disease, usually occupies only a relatively minor portion of the entire pathology section, and screening the area of interest is a tedious and time-consuming task. In this paper, deep learning techniques to investigate the pathological images of eyelid tumors. Inspired by the knowledge distillation process, we propose the Multiscale-Attention-Crop-ResNet (MAC-ResNet) network model to achieve the automatic classification of three malignant tumors and the automatic localization of whole slide imaging (WSI) lesion regions using U-Net. The final accuracy rates of the three classification problems of eyelid tumors on MAC-ResNet were 96.8%, 94.6%, and 90.8%, respectively.

Keywords: deep learning; eyelid tumor classification; digital pathology images; MAC-ResNet

Citation: Huang, X.; Yao, C.; Xu, F.; Chen, L.; Wang, H.; Chen, X.; Ye, J.; Wang, Y. MAC-ResNet: Knowledge Distillation Based Lightweight Multiscale-Attention-Crop-ResNet for Eyelid Tumors Detection and Classification. *J. Pers. Med.* **2023**, *13*, 89. https://doi.org/10.3390/jpm13010089

Academic Editor: Jiawei Zhou

Received: 23 November 2022
Revised: 21 December 2022
Accepted: 22 December 2022
Published: 29 December 2022

1. Introduction

Eyelid tumors are complicated and diverse, including tumors of the eyelid, conjunctiva, various layers of ocular tissues (cornea, sclera, uvea, and retina), and ocular appendages (lacrimal apparatus, orbit, and periorbital tissues) [1–3]. Primary malignant tumors of the eye can spread to the periorbital area, intracranially or metastasize systematically, and malignant tumors of other organs and tissues throughout the body can also metastasize to the eye. Therefore, eyelid tumors cover almost all histological types of tumors in the whole body and are widely representative, which can be the best thing object of study for pathological diagnosis of tumors.

Basal cell carcinoma (BCC) is a type of skin cancer that originates in the basal cells of the epidermis. It is the most common type of skin cancer, often occurring on sun-exposed areas of the body. Meibomian gland carcinoma (MGC) is a rare form of cancer affecting the meibomian glands in the eyelid, which secrete an oily substance for eye lubrication. MGC typically presents as a slow-growing lump on the eyelid, potentially mistaken for a benign cyst. Cutaneous melanoma (CM) is a type of skin cancer arising from pigment-producing cells known as melanocytes. It is less common than BCC, but more aggressive and capable of spreading to other parts of the body if left untreated. CM typically appears as a dark-colored new or changing mole or patch of skin, but may also present as a pink or red patch. According to morbidity studies, BCC is the most common malignant eyelid tumor, followed by CM and MGC [4–7].

Computed Tomography (CT) and Magnetic Resonance Imaging (MRI) have their limitations that affect their respective clinical applications. A biopsy is an important tool for physicians to finally diagnose eyelid tumors, and pathological diagnosis is the "gold standard" of diagnosis, and observation and analysis of histopathological images of biopsies is an important basis for physicians to formulate the best treatment plan [8–10]. The observation and analysis generally require qualitative, localization, and scoping judgments. However, the extreme shortage of human resources and overload in pathology departments are far from meeting the needs of clinical patients for accurate and efficient diagnostic pathology. Accurate diagnosis of BCC, MGC, and CM is essential for optimal patient outcomes, as early diagnosis is a key factor in determining the likelihood of a cure. While the physical appearance of these skin cancers may be distinctive, a biopsy is typically required for definitive diagnosis. Histologically, these types of eyelid tumors can be similar, making it possible to misdiagnose based on histological slides alone. The importance of accurate diagnosis cannot be overstated, as 90% of patient survival has been associated with early detection in cases where pathology-based diagnosis is involved.

Inspired by the concept of knowledge distillation [11], we have trained a teacher-student model to classify and segment eyelid tumors with good performance and a smaller, more efficient student network. In this paper, we will study the classification and segmentation of tumors based on meaningful learning methods using eyelid tumor pathology images, and the overall flowchart of the network is shown in Figure 1. The main contribution of this paper includes the following points:

1. Propose the network model called Multiscale-Attention-Crop-ResNet (MAC-ResNet). This network model can achieve 96.8%, 94.6%, and 90.8% accuracy in automatically classifying three ocular malignancies, respectively.
2. By training the student network ResNet with MAC-ResNet as the teacher network with the help of the knowledge distillation method, we made the smaller-scale network model to obtain better classification results on the eyelid tumor dataset, which called ZLet dataset.
3. We train three targeted segmentation networks for each of the three different malignant tumors, which enable us to segment the corresponding tumor locations well. With the help of the classification and segmentation networks, we diagnose the disease and the rapid localization of the lesion area.

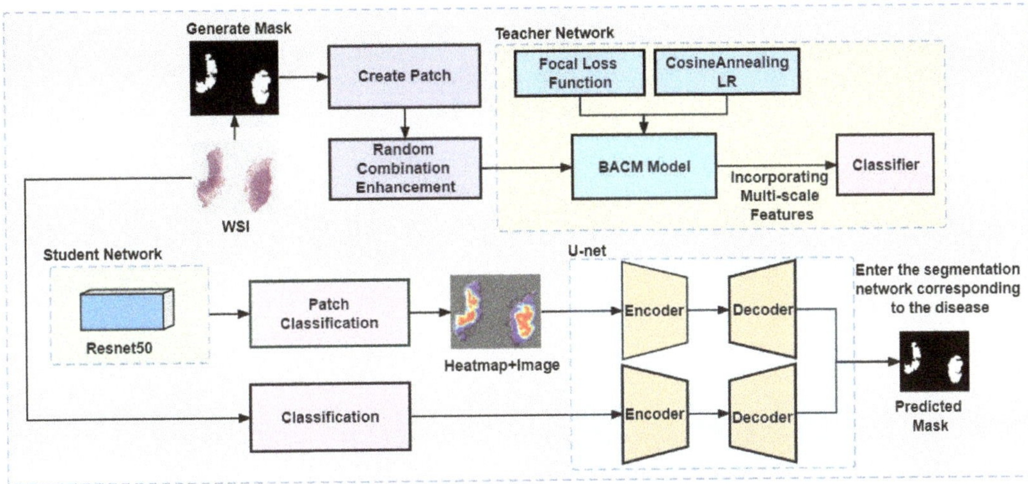

Figure 1. General flow-chart: the data were augmented using random combinatorial data processing; we proposed Mac-ResNet and used knowledge distillation to streamline the network. In addition, three segmentation networks were trained to learn the knowledge of three diseases and input to the corresponding class of segmentation networks to achieve the diagnosis of diseases as well as fast localization of lesion regions.

2. Related Work

The pathology segmentation and classification of eyelid tumors is a crucial aspect of ocular oncology as early diagnosis and treatment can significantly improve patient outcomes. One of the most common types of skin cancer that can occur on the eyelid is basal cell carcinoma (BCC). This type of cancer arises from the basal cells in the skin and is often caused by prolonged exposure to ultraviolet radiation. While BCC is not typically life-threatening, if left untreated it can cause significant damage to the skin and surrounding tissues. Cutaneous melanoma (CM), on the other hand, is a more aggressive form of skin cancer that originates from the pigment-producing cells in the skin. While less common than BCC, it has a higher likelihood of spreading to other parts of the body and can be deadly if not caught early. A rare type of cancer that can affect the eyelid is meibomian gland carcinoma (MGC), which arises from the meibomian glands that produce oil to keep the eye moist. MGC is generally more aggressive than BCC and can spread to other parts of the body if not treated promptly.

Accurately distinguishing between these three types of tumors is vital for treatment planning and research. Patients diagnosed with BCC may be treated with surgical or other local interventions to remove the tumor, while those diagnosed with cutaneous melanoma may require more aggressive treatment approaches, such as surgery, radiation therapy, or chemotherapy, in order to prevent the spread of the cancer. In addition, accurate classification and segmentation of eyelid tumors has significant value for research, including the study of the biology and genetics of these tumors, the evaluation of treatment response and disease progression, and the development of diagnostic and treatment algorithms. Therefore, a reliable method for classifying and segmenting eyelid tumors is necessary.

In recent years, with the development of deep learning in the field of computer vision, the study of medical image processing based on deep learning has become a popular research topic in the field of computer-aided diagnosis [12–14], and methods using deep learning are gradually being used for the diagnosis and screening of a variety of ophthalmic diseases, however, less research has been conducted on eyelid tumors.

In 2019, Hekler et al. will use a pre-trained ResNet50 [15] Network for training 695 whole slide images (WSIs) by migration learning to reduce the diagnosis error of benign moles and malignant melanoma [16]. Xie et al. used the VGG19 [17] network and ResNet50 network to classify patches generated from histopathological images [18]. In 2022 Wei Wen Hsu et al. proposed CNN for the classification of glioma subtypes using mixed data of WSIs and mpMRIs under weakly supervised learning [19], Nancy et al. proposed DenseNet-II [20] model through HAM10000 data set and various deep learning models to improve the accuracy of melanoma detection. At the 2018 ICCV conference, Chan et al proposed the HistoSegNet method for semantic segmentation of tissue types, using an annotated digital pathology atlas (ADP) for patched training, computation of gradient-weighted class activation maps, which outperforms other more complex weakly supervised semantic segmentation methods [21]. X Wang et al. based on the idea of model integration designed two complementary models based on SKM and scSEM to extract features from different spaces and scales, the method can directly segment the patches of digital pathology images pixel by pixel and no longer depends on the classification model [22].

Although computer vision has made some progress in the field of tumor segmentation, automated analysis studies based on eyelid tumor pathology are very rare due to the lack of dataset. In 2018, Ding et al. designed a study using CNN for the binary classification of malignant melanoma (MM) and the whole slide image-level classification was realized using a random forest classifier to assist pathologists in diagnosis [23]. In 2020, Wang et al. trained CNN on patch-level classification and used malignant probability to embed patches into each WSI to generate visualized heatmaps and also established a random forest model to establish WSI-level diagnosis [24]. Y Luo et al. performed patch prediction by a network model based on the DenseNet-161 architecture and WSI differentiation by an integration module based on the average probability strategy to differentiate between eyelid BCC and sebaceous carcinoma (SC) [25]. Parajuli et al. proposed a novel fully automated framework, including the use of DeeplabV3 for WSIs segmentation and the use of pre-trained VGG16 model, among others, to identify melanocytes and keratinocytes and support the diagnosis of melanoma [26]. Ye et al. first proposed a Cascade network to use the features from both histologic pattern and cellular atypia in a holistic pattern to detect and recognize malignant tumors in pathological slices of eyelid tumors with high accuracy [27]. Most of the above studies are based on existing methods and do not make significant modifications to the segmentation network. Some studies only focus on the recognition task and assist doctors in the diagnosis through classification, without involving tumor region segmentation due to the lack of a large-scale segmentation dataset in this task. Segmentation task is an important factor in evaluating the tumor stage and is also the basis for quantitative analysis. Our proposed method is able to simultaneously perform eyelid tumor classification and segmentation tasks based on histology slides through the design of the network architecture.

There are various factors that can increase the complexity of segmenting BCC, CM, and MGC in histology slides. The subtle differences in appearance that these tumors may exhibit compared to normal tissue, which can make them difficult to distinguish. Additionally, early-stage cancers may be more challenging to detect due to their small size and potential lack of discernible differences from normal tissue. To address these issues, we proposed the MAC-ResNet based on the teacher-student model for accurate classification and segmentation of eyelid tumors.

The teacher-student model is a machine learning paradigm in which a model, referred to as the "teacher", is trained to solve a task and then another model, referred to as the "student", is trained to mimic the teacher's behavior and solve the same task. The student model is typically trained on a smaller dataset and with fewer resources (e.g., fewer parameters or lower computational power) than the teacher, with the goal of achieving similar or improved performance at a lower cost.

The teacher-student model is also known as the knowledge distillation or model compression approach. It is often used to improve the efficiency and performance of machine learning models, particularly when deploying them in resource-constrained environments such as mobile devices or Internet of Things (IoT) devices. In the teacher-student model, the teacher model is first trained on a large dataset and then used to generate "soft" or "distilled" labels for the student model, which are more informative than the one-hot labels typically used for training. The student model is then trained using these soft labels and the original dataset, with the goal of learning to mimic the teacher's behavior. There are several variations of the teacher-student model, which can be divided into logits method distillation and feature distillation based on the transfer method. In this study, we adopt the logits method distillation. The concept of knowledge distillation and teacher-student model first appeared in "Distilling the knowledge in a neural network" by Hinton et al., and was used in image classification. Later, knowledge distillation was widely used in various fields of computer vision, such as face recognition [28], image/video segmentation [29], etc. In addition, it has also been applied in natural language processing (NLP) fields such as text generation [30], question answering systems [31], and others. Furthermore, it has also been applied in areas such as speech recognition [32] and recommender systems [33]. Finally, knowledge distillation has also been widely used in medical image processing. Qin et al. proposed a new knowledge distillation architecture in [34], achieving an improvement of 32.6% on the student network. Thi Kieu Khanh Ho et al. proposed a self-training KD framework in [35], achieving student network AUC improvements of up to 6.39%. However, this is the first time that knowledge distillation has been used in the classification of dermatopathology images.

3. Methods

First, we normalize and standardize the input data features and use a random combination image processing method to perform image expansion and enhancement. Then, we newly proposed a network structure (MAC-ResNet) that performs well on the classification task on the ZLet dataset, but the whole model structure is complex, consumes a lot of computational resources throughout the training process, and the speed of algorithm inference is slow. Therefore, we adopt the model compression method of knowledge distillation, use MAC-ResNet as the teacher network and ResNet50 as the student network, and achieve good results of the small volume student network ResNet50 in the classification of digital pathological pictures of eyelid tumors by using the knowledge of the teacher network to guide the training of the student network. Thus, this paper achieves automatic classification of three types of malignant tumors and enables automatic localization of lesion areas using U-Net [36].

3.1. MAC-ResNet

To solve the problem of low accuracy of fine-grained classification, we first propose the Watching-Smaller-Attention-Crop-ResNet (WSAC-ResNet) structure. It combines the Backbone-Attention-Crop-Model (BACM) module, the residual nested structure Double-Attention-Res-block, the SPP-block module, and the SampleInput module.

For the fine-grained classification problem, this paper refers to the fine-grained classification model WSDAN [37] and modifies it to design the Backbone-Attention-Crop-Model (BACM) module. From Figure 2, we can learn that the BACM Model consists of three parts. They are the backbone network, the attention module [38], and the AttentionPicture generated by cropping the original image according to the AttentionMap.

We crop and upsampling key regions of the images to a certain size according to the attention parameters, aiming to guide data for enhancement through the attention mechanism. Before the Feature Map of the neural network is input to the fully connected layer, it is input to the Attention model, and X Attention maps are obtained by convolution, dimensionality reduction, and other operations, each Attention map represents a feature in the picture, and one Attention map is randomly selected among the X Attention maps Then the normalization operation is performed on the Attention map. The normalization operation is as (1).

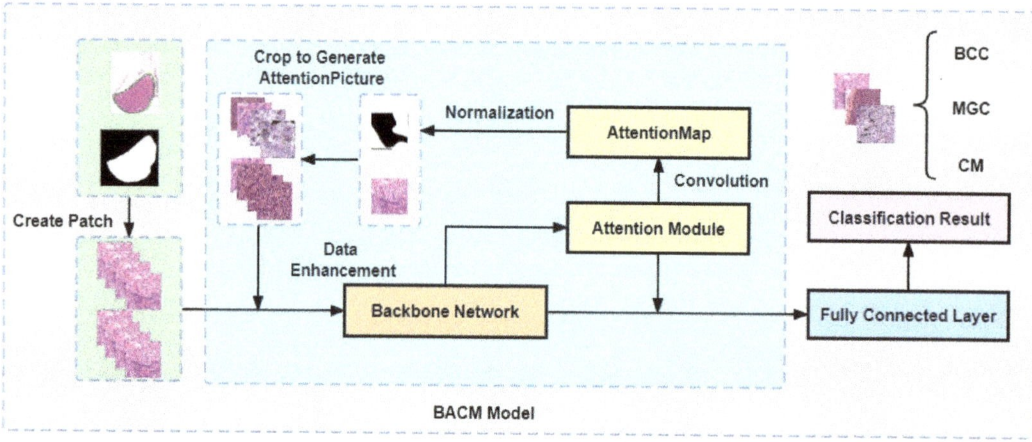

Figure 2. Details of BACM Model: This Network is referenced from the fine-grained classification model WSDAN and modified on its basis. The backbone network migrates the trained network parameters of the Imagenet dataset as the initial values of the network parameters.

$$A_k^* = (A_k - \min(A_k))/(\max(A_k) - \min(A_k)) \quad (1)$$

The value of the newly obtained Attention map is changed to 1 for elements with values more significant than the threshold θ_c and set to 0 for elements at other locations to generate a mask of locations worthy of strategic attention. The original image is cropped according to the generated mask against the original image to get the image of important regions and upsampling to a certain size, and then re-input into the neural network after data enhancement processing. When calculating the loss of the network model, the mean of the predicted and labeled loss of the original image and the predicted and labeled loss after cropping and re-inputting into the model is seen as the ultimate loss.

The backbone network is a neural network based on ResNet50 with a modified input structure named SampleInput, specifically by replacing a 7*7 convolutional layer with three 3*3 convolutional layers to enhance the network depth and ensure they have the same perceptual field; the network uses a double-layer nested residual structure Double-Attention-Res-block (DARes-block), which can fuse the deep layer with the shallow layer and the feature maps of the middle layer; SPP-block, which originated from SPPNet [39], is used to solve the training problem for different image sizes.

To further improve the classification of the network, the loss function and the learning rate adjustment strategy of this network will be optimized.

For the classification of unbalanced samples, the focal loss function [40] is used, which is a modification of the cross-entropy loss function, as (2).

$$FL(p_t) = -a_t(1 - p_t)^\gamma \log(p_t) \quad (2)$$

We use CosineAnnealingLR [41] to adjust the learning rate. It is used to change the magnitude of the learning rate by the cosine function, and each time the minimum point is reached. The next step resets the value of the learning rate to the maximum value to start a new round of decay.

We named the network that uses the above modules and policies as Multiscale-Attention-Crop-ResNet (MAC-ResNet).

3.2. Network Optimization Based On Knowledge Distillation

First, the teacher network with a complex model and good performance is trained, then the trained teacher network guides the training of the student network, and the trained student network is used to classify the dataset [42]. The main principle of the teacher network guiding the training of the student network is that the soft labels output by the teacher network and the output of the soft label by the student network are combined to coach the student network to complete the training of the hard labels (as shown in Figure 3). Soft labeling means that the predicted output of the network is divided by the temperature coefficient T and then the softmax operation is performed, which makes the result values between 0 and 1 with a more moderate distribution of values, while hard labeling means that the predicted output of the network is directly softmaxed without dividing by T [43].

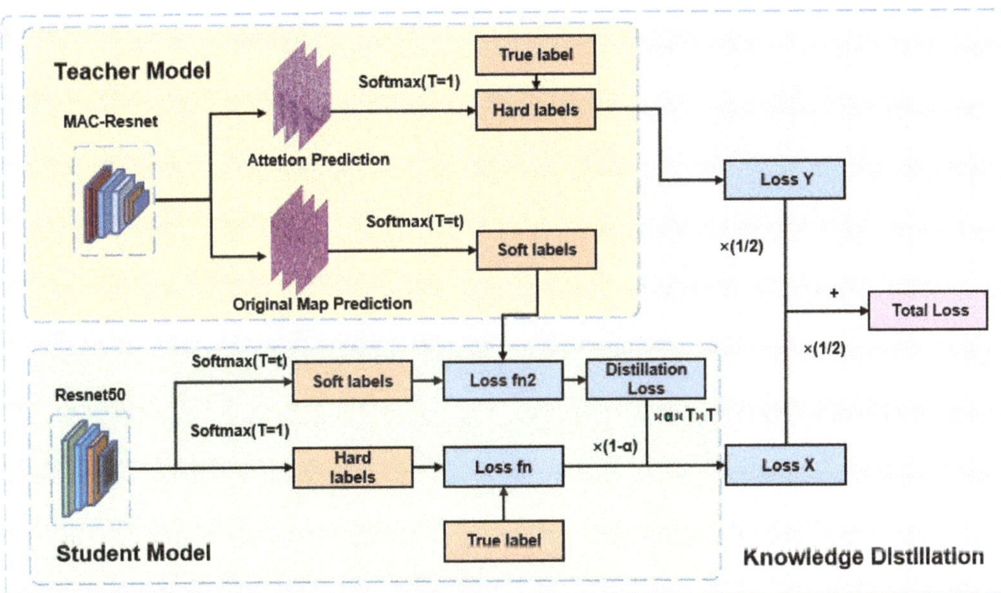

Figure 3. Details of Knowledge Distillation: MAC-ResNet is used as the teacher network to guide the training of student network ResNet, and the simplified network can also achieve better classification effects in the ZLet dataset.

Traditional segmentation networks consume a large amount of computing resources during the entire training process and has a slow inference speed during the training of large pathology dataset. It is possible to compress the segmentation model to generate a smaller network with similar performance. We adopt the model compression method of knowledge distillation, using the aforementioned MAC-ResNet as the teacher network. Then, we use the simple and classic ResNet50 as the student network. Finally, we achieve good classification results on the ocular tumor pathology image dataset using the relatively simple student network. Knowledge distillation is a method proposed by Hinton et al. [42], in which a complex and large model is used as the Teacher model, while the student model has a simpler structure. The Teacher model assists in the training of the student model, which has weaker learning ability, by transferring the knowledge it has learned to the student model, thereby enhancing the Student model's generalization ability. Therefore, in the knowledge distillation process, the teacher network is usually a network with a complex structure, slow inference process, high consumption of computer resources, and good model performance, while the student network is usually a network with a simpler structure, fewer parameters, and poorer model performance. The process of using knowledge distillation is as follows: first, we train the complex and well-performing teacher network (MAC-ResNet), then guide the training of the student network (ResNet50) using the trained teacher network, and finally use the trained student network to classify the dataset. The teacher network guides the training of the student network by providing the student network with soft labels, or the probabilities of each class predicted by the teacher network, instead of hard labels (as shown in Figure 3), which is the one-hot encoded labels of each class. For soft labeling, the predicted output of the network is divided by the temperature coefficient T and then the softmax operation is performed, which makes the result values between 0 and 1 with a more moderate distribution of values, while hard labeling means that the predicted output of the network is directly softmaxed without dividing by T [43]. This helps the student network learn from the rich information provided by the teacher network. The softmax process can be denote as:

$$\text{Softmax}(T) = (\exp(z_i/T))/\left(\sum_j \exp(z_i/T)\right) \tag{3}$$

The loss of the MAC-ResNet network consists of two parts, which are the loss between the predicted value and the label of the first original input picture and the loss between the predicted value and the label of the network model after the attention-guided cropping to generate AttentionPicture into the network, and the weighted sum between them is the final loss. The proposed loss function of the whole training process after using MAC-ResNet as the teacher network and ResNet50 as the student network is shown in (4) and (5).

$$\text{L}_{KD} = (1-a)\,\text{L}_f(\text{S}_{HP}, \text{label}) + (\text{a} * T * T)L_1(\text{S}_{SP}, \text{T}_{SL}) \tag{4}$$

$$\text{T}_{loss} = 1/2 * \text{L}_{KD} + 1/2 * \text{L}_f(\text{T}_{AHP}, \text{label}) \tag{5}$$

where S_{SP} refers to the output of the hard label by the student network, S_{SP} refers to the output of the soft label by the student network, T_{SL} refers to the soft labels generated by the teacher network for the original picture prediction, and T_{AHP} refers to the hard labels predicted by the teacher network based on the AttentionPicture (the labels are softened only for the results of the original picture prediction). Besides,L_{KD} refers to the loss of Knowledge Distillation, and T_{loss} refers to the total loss. L_1 is the K_L scattering loss function (Kullback-Leibler divergence), L_f is the focal loss function. T is the temperature coefficient, the larger the temperature coefficient, the more uniform the output data distribution.

After using knowledge distillation, the lightweight network model ResNet50, which is a student network, showed a significant improvement in the classification of the ZLet dataset

4. Experiment and Result

4.1. Data and Process

4.1.1. Data Gathering

We collected an eyelid tumor segmentation dataset, ZJU-LS eyelid tumor (ZLet) dataset, including 728 whole slide images and corresponding tumor masks. This is the largest eyelid tumor dataset ever reported. Over a period of seven years from January 2014 to January 2021, we collected pathological tissue slides from 132 patients treated at the Second Affiliated Hospital, Zhejiang University School of Medicine (ZJU-2) and Lishui Municipal Central Hospital (Lishui). We then used hematoxylin and eosin (H&E) staining to visualize the components and general morphological features of the tissue slides, enabling pathologists to observe and annotate them. Finally, we used KF-PRO-005 (KFBio, Zhejiang, China) to digitally amplify all pathological tissue slides at 20× magnification, resulting in a total of 728 whole slide images, including 136 BCC, 111 MGC, and 481 CM, as shown in the figure. These fully-annotated WSI were observed, diagnosed, and labeled by three experienced pathologists (>5000 h experience). The area marked by the doctors only contained the tumor of that category. To facilitate deep learning, we divided these

WSI into training, validation, and testing sets. The training set included 425 CM, 124 BCC, and 81 MGC. The validation set included 48 CM, 12 BCC, and 9 MGC. The testing set included 8 CM, 21 BCC, and 21 MGC. Some examples are demonstrate in Figure 4.

(a)Class Distribution

Class	Cutaneous Melanoma	Basal Cell Carcinoma	Meibomian Gland Carcinoma
Images	481	136	111

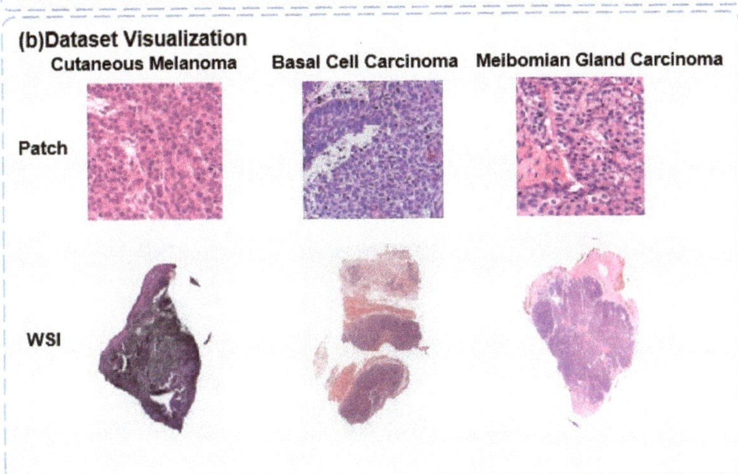

Figure 4. Details of Dataset: (**a**) denotes the class distribution and the number of images in the ZLet dataset, and (**b**) represents the data visualization of each type of eyelid tumor.

4.1.2. Data Preprocessing

During training, to decrease the need for memory and speed up the training process, we divided the full-field digital slices into small blocks based on the diseased regions labeled by the physician and then cropped the diseased regions. When generating the patch, the mask image is compared with the pathology image, and we crop the pathology image area corresponding to the white area of the mask image, the size of the crop is 512×512, stride = 256, which means there is an overlap of the image to crop. If the diseased area(the area with the value of 1 in the mask) in the current clipping area is more than 3/4 of the total area, the patch is kept, otherwise, it is discarded. The purpose of this is to prevent the patch from containing only a small number of diseased regions. After obtaining all the tiny patches, the cropped data were cleaned of images smaller than 330 kb, because images smaller than 330 kb in size contain a small number of scattered tissue regions, and such images can interfere with the training of the neural network. We also normalized and standardized the data features before feeding them into the neural network.

4.1.3. Data Augmentation

Before a batch of images is input to the neural network, we randomly select random flips, random rotations, horizontal flips, and vertical flips, modify the saturation of the image, add Gaussian noise, extract the outline of the image, and finally apply a combination of smoothing operations on the image, so that the same image in different training batches will generate many different transformed images, and the operation can be performed faster to get The enhanced results are obtained faster and do not require additional storage space to store the images. This operation not only enriches the data input to the neural network but also increases the features of the data, allowing the neural network to learn more features and enhancing the generalization ability of the model.

4.2. Ablation Study

To explore the effect of having the nested residual module DARes-block in different positions in ResNet50 on the experimental results, we designed an experiment keeping the original input unchanged and using the network structure of ResNet50+BACM. Table 1 shows the best results on the validation set for each group of experiments using DARes-block for the network structure in this chapter, where ACC denotes accuracy, Spec denotes specificity, Recall denotes recall, and 0-ACC is the accuracy of class 0.

Table 1. Validation set results of comparative experiments using the location of the DARes-block module.

DARes-Block Usage Location	ACC	Spec	Recall	0-ACC	1-ACC	2-ACC	3-ACC
layer2	0.8020	0.8244	0.7630	0.8672	0.7082	0.7306	0.8807
layer3	0.8110	0.8207	0.7800	0.8774	0.7150	0.7370	0.8954
layer4	0.8172	**0.8369**	0.7714	0.8858	0.7271	0.7493	0.8860
layer2 + layer3	0.8065	0.8243	0.7697	0.8695	0.7231	0.7462	0.8876
layer2 + layer4	**0.8307**	0.847	**0.8030**	**0.8873**	0.7456	**0.7785**	**0.8930**
layer3 + layer4	0.8261	0.8260	0.7963	0.8689	**0.7590**	0.78	0.8965
layer2 + layer3 + layer4	0.8187	0.8207	0.7815	0.8595	0.7476	0.7764	0.8911

From Table 1, we can see that the use of DARes-Block improves t network performance whether the modified residual structure block DARes-Block is used in layer2, layer3, and layer4 separately or in the combination of layer2, layer3, and layer4. One of the best experimental results is the experiment using DARes-Block in both layer2 and layer4 structures. Through our analysis, we determine that it is because using the DARes-Block structure in layer4 enables us to obtain more detailed features. These features were then fed directly into the attention mechanism without going through other convolutional or pooling layers. Although an experiment used the DARes-Block structure in each layer, the experimental results were not the best because using the structure in each layer increases the complexity of the model and is prone to overfitting problems, resulting in poor test results. At the same time, we also found that the accuracy of all four categories improved after using the DARes-Block structure, and it is no longer obvious to focus on one category, which indicates that the structure is effective in fine-grained classification.

The next step is to explore the effect of modifying the input module on the network performance based on the addition of the residual structure block DARes-Block network structure at layer2+layer4.

Table 2 shows the experimental results for the network with or without modifying the input module, which are the best results for each group of experiments on the validation set.

Table 2. Validation set results for comparison tests using modified input modules.

Whether to Modify the Input	ACC	Spec	Recall	0-ACC	1-ACC	2-ACC	3-ACC
NO	0.8307	0.8470	0.8030	0.8873	0.7456	0.7785	0.8930
YES	**0.8321**	**0.8739**	**0.8140**	**0.8901**	**0.7489**	**0.7857**	**0.9035**

The accuracy of the test set was improved somewhat by modifying the input structure on the ResNet50+BACM+DARes-Block network model structure from Table 2 above, but the improvement was not too significant. Since the modification of the input module did not cause a considerable increase in network complexity and did not additionally increase the training time of the network, we kept the modified input module.

Then, to investigate the role of SPP-Block, we designed the experiments still using the control variable method. The difference between the experiments is whether the SPP-

Block module is used; both are network structures with modified input structures on the ResNet50+BACM+DARes-Block model structure, except for this difference.

From the comparison experiments in Table 3, we can see that the model's performance is slightly improved with the SPP-block than without this structure, indicating that the SPP-block is beneficial for improving the model's performance. Ultimately, we refer to the structure using the above modification as WSAC-ResNet.

Table 3. Comparative experimental results of SPP-block.

	ACC	Spec	Recall	0-ACC	1-ACC	2-ACC	3-ACC
Without SPP-block	0.8321	0.8739	0.8140	0.8901	**0.7489**	0.7857	0.9035
With SPP-block	**0.8389**	**0.8792**	**0.8260**	**0.9135**	0.7407	**0.7914**	**0.9100**

To verify the effect of different loss functions on the classification effect of WSAC-ResNet, we designed experiments to compare the effect of three different loss functions on the classification effect. The experiments were conducted using the control variables method, and the three sets were identical except for the loss function, which used the same WSAC-ResNet network structure and parameters as the previous experiments. When using Focal loss, the values of and are set as default values, and the smoothing factor is set to 0.1, and the results of the experiment with the best effect on the validation set are also taken in the comparison experiment.

Figure 5 shows the comparison of the loss of the WSAC-ResNet network model during training using different loss functions. Among them, Labelsmoothing mitigates the overfitting problem by a regularization method that adds noise and reduces the weight of the true label in calculating the loss [44]. The loss values are recorded at 2 intervals during training. In this iterative analysis of the training losses for focal loss, cross-entropy loss, and label loss, it was observed that the focal loss initially started at a value of 1.8, but quickly dropped to 1.0 after about 200 steps. The cross-entropy loss, on the other hand, remained relatively stable at a value of around 1.4, while the label loss was the highest of the three losses at the beginning, but dropped to the middle of the other two losses after about 200 steps. After 500 steps, the three losses seemed to stabilize, with focal loss remaining at 0.66, label loss stable at 0.74, and cross-entropy loss staying at 0.85. This pattern of loss values suggests that the model may be more sensitive to the focal loss and may be learning more effectively using this loss function compared to the other two loss functions. Due to the uneven distribution of data among different classes and the inability of the labeled tags to be totally accurate, focal loss has an advantage both in terms of training time and performance.

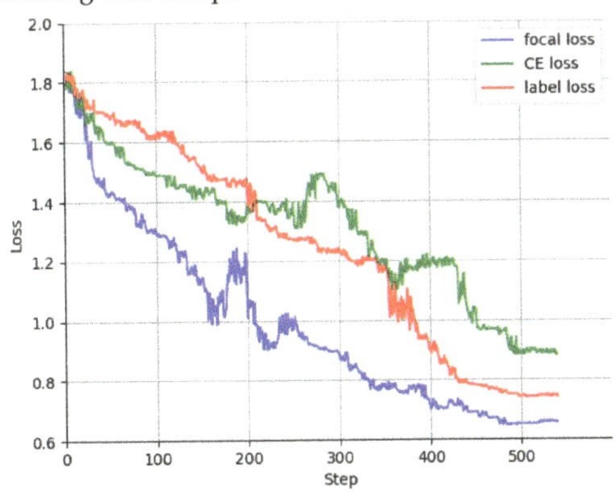

Figure 5. Comparative experimental results of the loss function. Due to the imbalance in classes, focal loss outcompetes other losses during the training process.

From the comparison in Table 4, we know that using focal loss is better than using Cross Entropy, label smoothing model, where the accuracy is improved by about 2% when using focal loss, and the accuracy of class 1 disease and class 2 disease is improved from 0.7858 and 0.826 to 0.862 and 0.871. The accuracy is improved by about 1% when using label smoothing. Observing the loss comparison graph, at the late loss convergence, the loss using focal loss is lower than that using Cross Entropy, and the label smoothing loss converges slower and at the early stage, the value of his loss is larger than that of both other approaches.

Table 4. Comparative experimental results of the loss function.

Loss Function	ACC	Spec	Recall	0-ACC	1-ACC	2-ACC	3-ACC
Cross Entropy	0.8646	0.8768	0.8522	0.9209	0.7858	0.8260	0.9257
Labelsmoothing	0.8704	0.8752	**0.8803**	**0.9200**	0.7892	0.8370	**0.9354**
Focal loss	**0.8857**	**0.8835**	0.8704	0.8945	**0.8620**	**0.8710**	0.9153

Therefore, both focal loss and label smoothing have improved the classification effect of WSAC-ResNet, but the WSAC-ResNet network model combined with the focal loss function is more effective because focal loss can alleviate the problem that the network model focuses on training a certain class due to the imbalance of dataset between classes. Therefore, the loss function of WSAC-ResNet is set to focal loss.

From Table 5 above and the previous experimental results, we can learn that the classification accuracy of the two strategies, focal loss and CosineAnnealingLR, when used in combination, reached 0.9023, naming the network model with the combination of WSAC-ResNet, focal loss, and CosineAnnealingLR as Multiscale- Attention-Crop-ResNet (MAC-ResNet).

Table 5. Comparison table of experimental results of WSAC-ResNet combination using optimized loss function and changing learning rate.

Loss	lr	ACC	Spec	Recall	0-ACC	1-ACC	2-ACC	3-ACC
CE	0.0001	0.8646	0.8768	0.8522	0.9209	0.7858	0.8260	0.9257
Focal loss	0.0001	0.8857	0.8835	0.8704	0.8945	0.8620	0.8710	0.9153
CE	CosineAnnealingLR	0.8805	0.8876	0.8692	**0.9310**	0.8176	0.8547	**0.9187**
Focal loss	CosineAnnealingLR	**0.9023**	**0.8992**	**0.9015**	0.9162	**0.8820**	**0.8937**	0.9175

4.3. *Preformance*

4.3.1. Network Training

Our experiments are based on the Pytorch. The experimental operating system is Ubuntu 20.04, With AMD R9 5950X, two NVIDIA 3080 10 GB graphic cards, and 128 GB of RAM. We trained our network from scratch for 50 epochs. The batch size is set to 8 for all experiments and a learning rate of 0.00001.

4.3.2. Evaluation Metrics

To evaluate the classification performance of our network, we used various evaluation metrics including Sensitivity, Specificity, and Accuracy. Also, we used two evaluation metrics, IOU and Dice, to evaluate the segmentation performance of our network. Their formulas are as follows:

$$\text{Sensitivity} = \frac{TP}{TP+FN} \tag{6}$$

$$\text{Specificity} = \frac{TN}{TN+FP} \tag{7}$$

$$\text{Accuracy} = \frac{TP+TN}{TP+TN+FP+FN} \tag{8}$$

$$\mathrm{IOU} = \frac{TP}{FN + TP + FP} \tag{9}$$

$$\mathrm{Dice} = \frac{2 \times TP}{FN + TP + TP + FP} \tag{10}$$

4.3.3. Patch-Level Classification

To demonstrate the performance of our model for the three eyelid tumor classification problems, we used the classical metrics sensitivity, specificity, and accuracy in the classification problem to measure the classification results. As shown in Table 6, the classification results for all three eyelid tumors are relatively high, which reflects the significant effectiveness of our model in the triple classification problem of eyelid tumors.

Table 6. Overall average classification results.

Eyelid Tumor	Sensitivity	Specificity	Accuracy
BCC	0.8046	0.9862	0.9688
MGC	0.7688	0.9589	0.9467
CM	0.8889	0.9113	0.9089

4.3.4. WSI-Level Results

At the WSI level, we segmented the classified and reorganized WSI map and the original WSI map with the traditional U-Net, and the results were combined to finally segment the focal regions of the three eyelid tumors. The segmentation results are shown in Table 7, and their metrics indicate that their method can meet the need for rapid determination of the lesion regions, and the segmented images are visualized as shown in the ground truth in Figure 6.

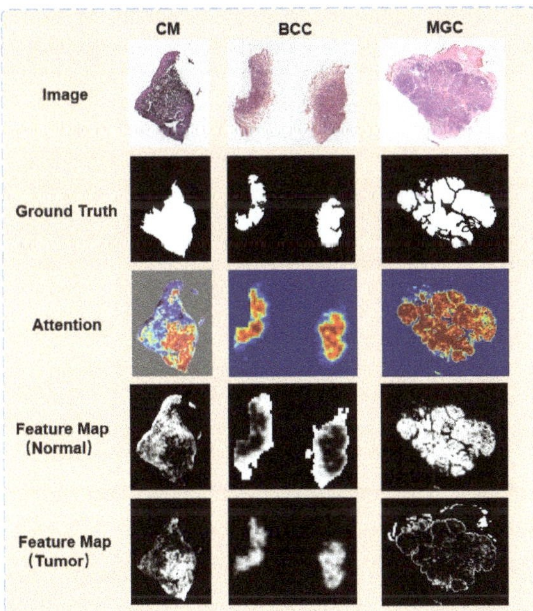

Figure 6. Visualization of results: The segmentation results can provide the doctor with aid in diagnosing what kind of tumor the pathology image contains and where the tumor is located.

Table 7. Overall average segmentation results.

Eyelid Tumor	IOU	Dice
BCC	0.7277	0.8349
MGC	0.6806	0.8050
CM	0.7329	0.8307

This segmentation result can suggest that the doctor should focus on this region, which has a high probability of having some kind of tumor and provide aid to the doctor to diagnose which kind of tumor the pathological image contains and where the tumor is located, which can help to remove the tumor later. In addition, the classification results on the patches can be combined to form an attention map, and by processing the attention map, we can get the feature maps of the model for the normal and tumor regions (as shown in Figure 6 the attention, feature map). These tumor feature maps can further help doctors to analyze the tumor in pathology slides, which is a reliable basis for doctors' diagnostic analysis.

5. Conclusions

The segmentation based on pathology slides is usually time consuming. In order to improve efficiency, we have adopted the knowledge distillation method, inspired by Hinton et al., to train a student network using a MAC-ResNet as the teacher network, enabling the student network to achieve good accuracy on the target task even with a small capacity. In addition, by using U-Net to achieve automatic localization of the lesion area, we can provide a reliable foundation for the diagnosis of pathologists and improve the efficiency and accuracy of diagnosis. We have applied this method to pathology tumor detection for the first time and have successfully verified the practicality of the teacher-student model in the field of pathology image analysis. Finally, the accuracy of MAC-ResNet on the three target tasks was 96.8%, 94.6%, and 90.8%, respectively. However, this study also had some regrets that we were not able to conduct extensive experiments on this data to widely verify the performance of different methods under the teacher-student framework. Another limitation of this study is that it only studied BCC, MGC, and CM, while eyelid tumors include other diseases, so more data sets will be needed in the future. We are currently working on a larger data set, ZLet-large, based on ZLet. ZLet-large includes over a thousand eyelid tumor pathology images and an increased number of disease types, including squamous cell carcinoma (SCC), seborrheic keratosis (SK), and xanthelasma. We hope to be able to conduct more extensive experiments on ZLet-large to further explore the potential of the teacher-student model in the analysis of eyelid tumors.

Author Contributions: Conceptualization, X.H. and C.Y.; data curation, C.Y.; writing—original draft preparation, F.X., L.C. and X.H.; writing—review and editing, Y.W., X.C. and J.Y.; visualization, H.W. All authors have read and agreed to the published version of the manuscript.

Funding: This research was supported in part by the National Natural Science Foundation of China (No. 62206242), and the National Natural Science Foundation of China (No. 2019YFC0118404).

Institutional Review Board Statement: Not applicable.

Informed Consent Statement: Not applicable.

Data Availability Statement: Not applicable.

Acknowledgments: The authors would like to thank the support from the Pathology Center of the Second Affiliated Hospital of Zhejiang University School of Medicine (ZJU-2) and the institutions that generously built the open-source dataset.

Conflicts of Interest: The authors declare no conflict of interest.

References

1. Singh, A.D.; Seregard, S. *Ocular Tumors*; Karger Medical and Scientific Publishers: Basel, Switzerland, 2016.
2. Shields, J.A.; Shields, C.L. Ocular Tumors of Childhood. *Pediatr. Clin. N. Am.* **1993**, *40*, 805–826.
3. Stannard, C.; Sauerwein, W.; Maree, G.; Lecuona, K. Radiotherapy for ocular tumours. *Eye* **2013**, *27*, 119–127.
4. Cook, B.E.; Bartley, G.B. Treatment options and future prospects for the management of eyelid malignancies: An evidence-based update. *Ophthalmology* **2001**, *108*, 2088–2098.
5. Rubin, A.I.; Chen, E.H.; Ratner, D. Basal-cell carcinoma. *N. Engl. J. Med.* **2005**, *353*, 2262–2269.
6. Slutsky, J.B.; Jones, E.C. Periocular Cutaneous Malignancies: A Review of the Literature. *Dermatol. Surg.* **2012**, *38*, 552–569.
7. Ohara, M.; Sotozono, C.; Tsuchihashi, Y.; Kinoshita, S. Ki-67 labeling index as a marker of malignancy in ocular surface neoplasms. *Jpn. J. Ophthalmol.* **2004**, *48*, 524–529.
8. Araújo, T.; Aresta, G.; Castro, E.; Rouco, J.; Aguiar, P.; Eloy, C.; Polónia, A.; Campilho, A. Classification of breast cancer histology images using Convolutional Neural Networks. *PLoS ONE* **2017**, *12*, e0177544.
9. Bardou, D.; Zhang, K.; Ahmad, S.M. Classification of Breast Cancer Based on Histology Images Using Convolutional Neural Networks. *IEEE Access* **2018**, *6*, 24680–24693.
10. Hu, H.; Qiao, S.; Hao, Y.; Bai, Y.; Cheng, R.; Zhang, W.; Zhang, G. Breast cancer histopathological images recognition based on two-stage nuclei segmentation strategy. *PLoS ONE* **2022**, *17*, e0266973.
11. Hinton, G.; Geoffrey, V.; Jeff, D. Distilling the knowledge in a neural network. *arXiv* **2015**, arXiv:1503.02531.
12. Fujisawa, Y.; Inoue, S.; Nakamura, Y. The Possibility of Deep Learning-Based, Computer-Aided Skin Tumor Classifiers. *Front. Med.* **2019**, *6*, 191.
13. De, A.; Sarda, A.; Gupta, S.; Das, S. Use of artificial intelligence in dermatology. *Indian J. Dermatol.* **2020**, *65*, 352.
14. Chen, S.B.; Novoa, R.A. Artificial intelligence for dermatopathology: Current trends and the road ahead. *Semin. Diagn. Pathol.* **2022**, *39*, 298–304.
15. He, K.; Zhang, X.; Ren, S.; Sun, J. Deep residual learning for image recognition. In Proceedings of the IEEE Conference on Computer Vision and Pattern Recognition (CVPR), Las Vegas, NV, USA, 27–30 June 2016; pp. 770–778.
16. Hekler, A.; Utikal, J.S.; Enk, A.H.; Berking, C.; Klode, J.; Schadendorf, D.; Jansen, P.; Franklin, C.; Holland-Letz, T.; Krahl, D.; et al. Pathologist-level classification of histopathological melanoma images with deep neural networks. *Eur. J. Cancer* **2019**, *115*, 79–83.
17. Simonyan, K.; Zisserman, A. Very deep convolutional networks for large-scale image recognition *arXiv* **2015**, arXiv:1409.1556.
18. Xie, P.; Zuo, K.; Zhang, Y.; Li, F.; Yin, M.; Lu, K. Interpretable classification from skin cancer histology slides using deep learning: A retrospective multicenter study. *arXiv* **2019**, arXiv:1904.06156.
19. Hsu, W.W.; Guo, J.M.; Pei, L.; Chiang, L.A.; Li, Y.F.; Hsiao, J.C.; Colen, R.; Liu, P. A weakly supervised deep learning-based method for glioma subtype classification using WSI and mpMRIs. *Sci. Rep.* **2022**, *12*, 6111.
20. Girdhar, N.; Sinha, A.; Gupta, S. DenseNet-II: An improved deep convolutional neural network for melanoma cancer detection. *Soft Comput.* **2022**, 1–20, doi:10.1007/s00500-022-07406-z.
21. Chan, L.; Hosseini, M.S.; Rowsell, C.; Plataniotis, K.N.; Damaskinos, S. HistoSegNet: Semantic Segmentation of Histological Tissue Type in Whole Slide Images. In Proceedings of the IEEE/CVF International Conference on Computer Vision (ICCV), Seoul, Republic of Korea, 27 October–2 November 2019; pp. 10661–10670.
22. Wang, X.; Fang, Y.; Yang, S.; Zhu, D.; Wang, M.; Zhang, J.; Tong, K.y.; Han, X. A hybrid network for automatic hepatocellular carcinoma segmentation in H&E-stained whole slide images. *Med Image Anal.* **2021**, *68*, 101914.
23. Ding, L.; Wang, L.; Huang, X.; Wang, Y.; Ye, J.; Sun, L. Deep learning-based accurate diagnosis of eyelid malignant melanoma from gigapixel pathologic slides. In Proceedings of the Tenth International Conference on Graphics and Image Processing (ICGIP 2018), Chengdu, China, 12–14 December 2018; Volume 11069, pp. 441–452.
24. Wang, L.; Ding, L.; Liu, Z.; Sun, L.; Chen, L.; Jia, R.; Dai, X.; Cao, J.; Ye, J. Automated identification of malignancy in whole-slide pathological images: Identification of eyelid malignant melanoma in gigapixel pathological slides using deep learning. *Br. J. Ophthalmol.* **2020**, *104*, 318–323.
25. Luo, Y.; Zhang, J.; Yang, Y.; Rao, Y.; Chen, X.; Shi, T.; Xu, S.; Jia, R.; Gao, X. Deep learning-based fully automated differential diagnosis of eyelid basal cell and sebaceous carcinoma using whole slide images. *Quant. Imaging Med. Surg.* **2022**, *12*, 4166–4175.
26. Parajuli, M.; Shaban, M.; Phung, T.L. Automated differentiation of skin melanocytes from keratinocytes in high-resolution histopathology images using a weakly-supervised deep-learning framework. *Int. J. Imaging Syst. Technol.* **2022**. https://doi.org/10.1002/ima.22810.
27. Ye, J.; Wang, L.; lv, D.; Wang, Y.; Chen, L.; Huang, Y.; Huang, F.; Ashraf, D.A.; Kersten, R.; Shao, A.; et al. *A Deep Learning Approach with Cascade-Network Design for Eyelid Tumors Diagnosis Based on Gigapixel Histopathology Images; Research Square* **2022**. https://doi.org/10.21203/rs.3.rs-1597378/v1.
28. Wang, X.; Fu, T.; Liao, S.; Wang, S.; Lei, Z.; Mei, T. Exclusivity-Consistency Regularized Knowledge Distillation for Face Recognition. In *Proceedings of the Computer Vision—ECCV 2020*; Vedaldi, A., Bischof, H., Brox, T., Frahm, J.M., Eds.; Springer International Publishing: Cham, Switzerland, 2020; pp. 325–342.
29. Hou, Y.; Ma, Z.; Liu, C.; Hui, T.W.; Loy, C.C. Inter-Region Affinity Distillation for Road Marking Segmentation. In Proceedings of the IEEE/CVF Conference on Computer Vision and Pattern Recognition (CVPR), Seattle, WA, USA, 2020.

30. Chen, Y.C.; Gan, Z.; Cheng, Y.; Liu, J.; Liu, J. Distilling Knowledge Learned in BERT for Text Generation. In Proceedings of the 58th Annual Meeting of the Association for Computational Linguistics, Online, 2020; pp. 7893–7905. https://doi.org/10.18653/v1/2020.acl-main.705.
31. Yang, Z.; Shou, L.; Gong, M.; Lin, W.; Jiang, D. Model Compression with Two-Stage Multi-Teacher Knowledge Distillation for Web Question Answering System. In Proceedings of the 13th International Conference on Web Search and Data Mining, Houston, TX, USA, 2020; Association for Computing Machinery: New York, NY, USA, 2020; pp. 690–698. https://doi.org/10.1145/3336191.3371792.
32. Shen, P.; Lu, X.; Li, S.; Kawai, H. Knowledge Distillation-Based Representation Learning for Short-Utterance Spoken Language Identification. *IEEE/ACM Trans. Audio, Speech, Lang. Process.* **2020**, *28*, 2674–2683. https://doi.org/10.1109/TASLP.2020.3023627
33. Chen, X.; Zhang, Y.; Xu, H.; Qin, Z.; Zha, H. Adversarial Distillation for Efficient Recommendation with External Knowledge *ACM Trans. Inf. Syst.* **2018**, *37*. https://doi.org/10.1145/3281659.
34. Qin, D.; Bu, J.J.; Liu, Z.; Shen, X.; Zhou, S.; Gu, J.J.; Wang, Z.H.; Wu, L.; Dai, H.F. Efficient Medical Image Segmentation Based on Knowledge Distillation. *IEEE Trans. Med Imaging* **2021**, *40*, 3820–3831. https://doi.org/10.1109/TMI.2021.3098703.
35. Ho, T.K.K.; Gwak, J. Utilizing Knowledge Distillation in Deep Learning for Classification of Chest X-Ray Abnormalities. *IEEE Access* **2020**, *8*, 160749–160761. https://doi.org/10.1109/ACCESS.2020.3020802.
36. Ronneberger, O.; Fischer, P.; Brox, T. *U-net: Convolutional Networks for Biomedical Image Segmentation*; Springer: Cham, Switzerland, 2015. pp. 234–241.
37. Hu, T.; Qi, H.; Huang, Q.; Lu, Y. See better before looking closer: Weakly supervised data augmentation network for fine-grained visual classification. *arXiv* **2019**, arXiv:1901.09891.
38. Mnih, V.; Heess, N.; Graves, A.; Kavukcuoglu, K. *Recurrent Models of Visual Attention; Advances in neural information processing systems* **2014**, *27*.
pp. 2204–2212.
39. He, K.; Zhang, X.; Ren, S.; Sun, J. Spatial pyramid pooling in deep convolutional networks for visual recognition. *IEEE Trans. Pattern Anal. Mach. Intell.* **2015**, *37*, 1904–1916.
40. Lin, T.Y.; Goyal, P.; Girshick, R.; He, K.; Dollár, P. Focal Loss for Dense Object Detection. *IEEE Trans. Pattern Anal. Mach. Intell.* **2020**, *42*, 318–327.
41. Loshchilov, I.; Hutter, F. SGDR: Stochastic Gradient Descent with Warm Restarts. *arXiv* **2017**, arXiv:1608.03983.
42. Gou, J.; Yu, B.; Maybank, S.J.; Tao, D. Knowledge distillation: A survey. *Int. J. Comput. Vis.* **2021**, *129*, 1789–1819.
43. Bridle, J. Training Stochastic Model Recognition Algorithms as Networks can Lead to Maximum Mutual Information Estimation of Parameters. In *Advances in Neural Information Processing Systems*; Touretzky, D., Ed.; Morgan-Kaufmann: Burlington, MA, USA 1989; Volume 2.
44. Szegedy, C.; Vanhoucke, V.; Ioffe, S.; Shlens, J.; Wojna, Z. Rethinking the inception architecture for computer vision. In Proceedings of the IEEE Conference on Computer Vision and Pattern Recognition, Las Vegas, NV, USA, 27–30 June 2016; pp. 2818–2826.

Journal of *Personalized Medicine*

MDPI

Article

End-to-End Deep-Learning-Based Diagnosis of Benign and Malignant Orbital Tumors on Computed Tomography Images

Ji Shao [1,†], Jiazhu Zhu [2,†], Kai Jin [1], Xiaojun Guan [3], Tianming Jian [4], Ying Xue [2], Changjun Wang [1], Xiaojun Xu [3], Fengyuan Sun [4], Ke Si [2], Wei Gong [2,*] and Juan Ye [1,*]

1 Department of Ophthalmology, The Second Affiliated Hospital of Zhejiang University, School of Medicine, Hangzhou 310009, China
2 Center for Neuroscience and Department of Neurobiology of the Second Affiliated Hospital, State Key Laboratory of Modern Optical Instrumentation, Zhejiang University School of Medicine, Hangzhou 310027, China
3 Department of Radiology, The Second Affiliated Hospital of Zhejiang University, School of Medicine, Hangzhou 310009, China
4 Tianjin International Joint Research and Development Centre of Ophthalmology and Vision Science, Eye Institute and School of Optometry, Tianjin Medical University Eye Hospital, Tianjin Medical University, Tianjin 300203, China
* Correspondence: weigong@zju.edu.cn (W.G.); yejuan@zju.edu.cn (J.Y.)
† These authors contributed equally to this work.

Abstract: Determining the nature of orbital tumors is challenging for current imaging interpretation methods, which hinders timely treatment. This study aimed to propose an end-to-end deep learning system to automatically diagnose orbital tumors. A multi-center dataset of 602 non-contrast-enhanced computed tomography (CT) images were prepared. After image annotation and preprocessing, the CT images were used to train and test the deep learning (DL) model for the following two stages: orbital tumor segmentation and classification. The performance on the testing set was compared with the assessment of three ophthalmologists. For tumor segmentation, the model achieved a satisfactory performance, with an average dice similarity coefficient of 0.89. The classification model had an accuracy of 86.96%, a sensitivity of 80.00%, and a specificity of 94.12%. The area under the receiver operating characteristics curve (AUC) of the 10-fold cross-validation ranged from 0.8439 to 0.9546. There was no significant difference on diagnostic performance of the DL-based system and three ophthalmologists ($p > 0.05$). The proposed end-to-end deep learning system could deliver accurate segmentation and diagnosis of orbital tumors based on noninvasive CT images. Its effectiveness and independence from human interaction allow the potential for tumor screening in the orbit and other parts of the body.

Keywords: hemangioma; lymphoma; deep learning; segmentation; classification

Citation: Shao, J.; Zhu, J.; Jin, K.; Guan, X.; Jian, T.; Xue, Y.; Wang, C.; Xu, X.; Sun, F.; Si, K.; et al. End-to-End Deep-Learning-Based Diagnosis of Benign and Malignant Orbital Tumors on Computed Tomography Images. *J. Pers. Med.* **2023**, *13*, 204. https://doi.org/10.3390/jpm13020204

Academic Editor: László Mangel

Received: 24 November 2022
Revised: 16 January 2023
Accepted: 22 January 2023
Published: 23 January 2023

1. Introduction

Early diagnosis of orbital tumors is critical for timely intervention, appropriate treatment selection, and prognosis prediction. Different orbital tumors have varying treatment protocols owing to their distinct cellular origins. Hemangioma is the most common primary benign orbital tumor, accounting for 6% of all orbital lesions [1]. It is characterized by slow growth [2]. Immediate surgical excision is only recommended in case of evident vision deterioration, while conservative treatment is a valid option for patients in the absence of vision deficits [3–5]. Contrastingly, radiotherapy is the first-line treatment for malignant lymphomas [6,7], which are the most common malignant neoplasms in adults [1,8]. The risk of malignant tumor metastases and recurrence increases without optimal clinical intervention, appropriate therapy protocol, and follow-up frequency. Therefore, the early diagnosis and timely treatment of orbital tumors are of crucial importance.

Computed tomography (CT) and magnetic resonance imaging (MRI) are the imaging modalities of choice for detecting orbital tumors [9,10]. Previously, ultrasound was a rapid, inexpensive, and non-invasive medical technology, but it is not the first choice for orbital tumor classification due to its limited value of size detection, location, and relationship to the surrounding structures [11]. CT and MRI are capable of providing images inside the orbit via radio waves and magnetic fields [12,13]. These techniques narrow the differential diagnosis and allow disease staging by assessing the tumor location, homogeneity, margin, signal intensity, and relationship with adjacent structures [10,14,15]. Compared with CT, MRI has an advantage in higher soft tissue resolution, but the application of orbital tumor screening is limited because of the expensive cost and long exam time. Contrast-enhanced CT and MRI could visualize blood flow in various types of orbital tumors, which is beneficial for diagnosing malignant and benign orbital tumors. However, contrast-enhanced CT and MRI are invasive technologies and cannot be performed on patients with contraindications, which include contrast agent allergy, renal insufficiency, claustrophobia, etc. [16]. All of these factors preclude the possibility of contrast-enhanced CT and MRI being well-suited orbital tumor screening tools. Non-contrast-enhanced CT is widely used for detecting orbital tumors, but the imaging findings often overlap and hence pose a diagnostic challenge [17].

Artificial intelligence (AI), a branch of computer science, represents the techniques that enable computers to simulate and extend human intelligence. Machine learning (ML) is a mainstream of AI technology, which is capable of automatically improving computer algorithms by analyzing the features of input rather than following explicit program instructions [18,19]. Conventional ML and deep learning (DL) are two variations of ML [20,21]. With the excellent ability to analyze high-level features, interpreting medical images based on DL has gradually become the research hotspot.

In recent years, DL has been paid increasing attention in the field of ophthalmology, and many DL-based models have been proposed to assist in the automatic diagnosis, grading, and prognosis prediction of various ocular diseases [22–24]. With the need for orbital image analysis skyrocketing, more and more DL networks have been applied to detect and segment intricate anatomical structures of the orbit [25,26]. The capability of achieving pixel-level classification on CT images using DL-based algorithms implies the potential for precise segmentation of orbital tumors. Previous studies had attempted to distinguish ocular adnexal lymphoma from idiopathic orbital inflammation on MRI images and reached diagnostic performance superior to the radiology resident [27,28]. DL-based models have also displayed outstanding performance for automatic tumor classification in medical imaging of multiple organs, such as the lung [29,30], brain [31], and breast [32]. Taken together, we hypothesized that DL-based algorithms had the efficacy of high-precision segmentation and classification of orbital tumors on CT images.

In this study, we retrospectively collected 602 non-contrast-enhanced CT images of 64 patients with orbital tumors (using cavernous hemangiomas and lymphomas as representatives of benign and malignant tumors) from two independent hospitals. An end-to-end DL-based model was established to automatically segment orbital tumors and distinguish malignant orbital tumors from benign ones.

2. Materials and Methods

2.1. Patients

This retrospective study was reviewed and approved by the institutional review board. All the patients enrolled in this study were recruited from two independent institutions: the Second Affiliated Hospital of Zhejiang University, from February 2009 to June 2020, and Tianjin Medical University Eye Hospital, from December 2017 to May 2018. The inclusion criteria were as follows: (1) histopathological diagnosis of hemangioma or lymphoma based on the excised tissues from the orbital lesions and (2) patients with non–contrast-enhanced CT images before surgery. The exclusion criteria were: (1) patients with unclear histopathological results; (2) poor CT image quality or without CT images in axial view; and (3) history of eye or orbital surgery, trauma, radiation treatment, or other orbital therapy.

2.2. CT Image Acquisition and Annotation

Non-contrast-enhanced CT scans (Sensation 16, Somatom perspective, Somatom Definition AS, and Somatom Definition Flash, Siemens Healthcare, Erlangen, Germany; Optima CT540, LightSpeed RT16, and ACTs, GE Healthcare, Milwaukee, USA) were performed on all patients with benign and malignant orbital tumors before surgical excision. The scanning parameters were as follows: 120–130 kVp, 180–300 mAs, 0.94 spiral pitch, and 1.0–4.0 mm slice thickness.

In all CT images, those showing orbital masses in the axial view were selected. A certified ophthalmologist with 2 years of experience used the ITK-SNAP software (version 3.6.0, www.itksnap.org, accessed on 21 January 2023) to manually annotate the ROI in each image. All labels were saved as TIFF images.

2.3. Preprocessing and Network Architecture

In this study, a total of 602 non-contrast-enhanced CT images from 64 patients were included, which were randomly divided into a training set with 482 images, a validation set with 51 images, and a testing set with 69 images. An end-to-end DL-based system composed of U-Net and ResNet-34 was established to detect and classify orbital tumors. We trained these two sub-networks independently and finally tested the entire system. Figure 1 illustrates the workflow of this study.

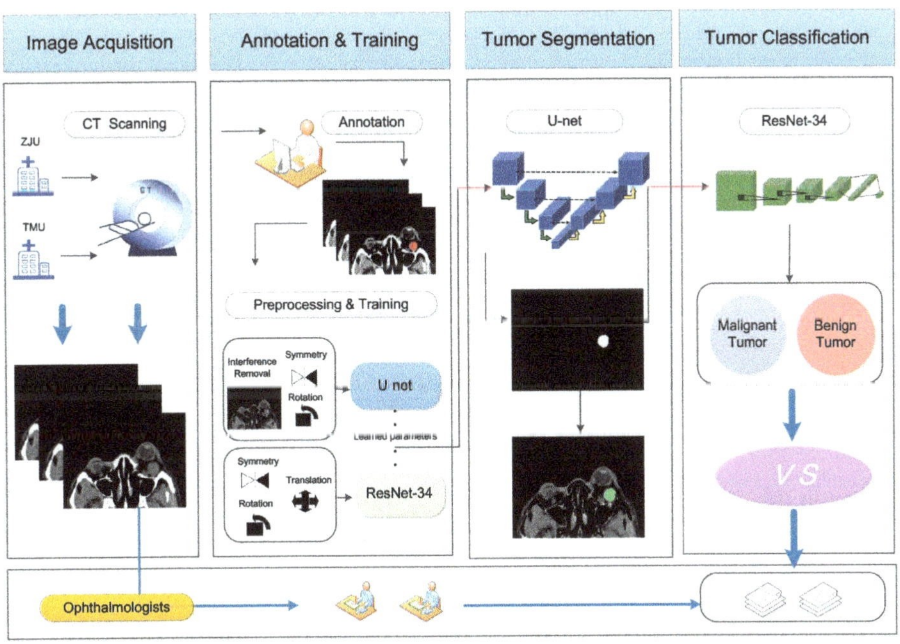

Figure 1. Workflow of the proposed method; CT, computed tomography.

2.3.1. Preprocessing of the CT Images

In the preprocessing step, the original CT images in the format of DICOM were converted into 512 × 512 grayscale images in the format of TIFF. To avoid misidentifying non-tumor tissue with high signals as orbital tumors, the grayscale values of all pixels with more than 200 were reset to zero. Then, to speed up the training process, the input images were resized to 256 × 256 resolution. The data augmentation technique was applied to solve the overfitting caused by the small dataset. Symmetry and rotation transformation (with a maximum rotation angle of 10°) were adopted in the U-Net training set. In the ResNet-34 training set, a translational transformation (horizontal and vertical) was used.

2.3.2. Segmentation Network

The automatic segmentation network was trained with U-Net as the backbone. U-Net is one of the most popular network structures in medical image segmentation, which shows advanced performance in the segmentation of small targets [33]. In this study, we used the non-contrast-enhanced orbital CT images to train a 2-dimensional U-Net for orbital tumor detection and segmentation. The U-Net, containing an encoder and a decoder, has a U-shaped structure. During the encoding stage, multi-scale feature maps are extracted from input images through multiple down-sampling. The size of the feature map decreased from 256×256 as input to 16×16 at the bottom, and the number of channels increased from 1 at the origin to 1024 at the last. Inversely, in the decoding stage, the up-sampling operation was conducted to sequentially recover high-level semantic information. Meanwhile, the low-level details of different scales at the down-sampling step were combined with the high-level semantics at the up-sampling step by skip connection, which was conducive to generating more accurate segmentation masks. The size of the feature map increased from 16×16 to 256×256, and the number of channels decreased from 1024 to 1. The output was a probability map of the orbital tumor. This probability map was binarized to get the mask images of orbital tumors, and the threshold was set to 0.5. The local tiny outliers were eliminated using a denoising approach to further enhance the segmentation performance. Additionally, the small cavities within the segmented orbital tumors were fulfilled by the morphological process. The final boundary of the segmented orbital tumor was smoothed using median filtering to approximate the shape of ground truth. Gradient descent was performed using the Adam optimizer, and cross entropy was employed to represent the loss function. The batch size was set to 2, and the epoch was set to 300. The initial learning rate was set to 0.001; then, every 80 epochs it was reduced by a factor of 10.

2.3.3. Classification Network

The classification network was based on ResNet-34 [34], which used 3×3 convolution kernels to extract high-level features of CT images through the deep structure. It was composed of an input convolutional layer, a max-pooling layer, 16 residual blocks, an average pooling layer, a fully connected layer, and a softmax layer. Each residual block consisted of two convolution layers and an identity mapping. Three of these residual blocks were special. Since the convolution layer changed the size of the feature map and the number of channels, the identity mapping additionally introduced the convolution kernel of 1×1 to reduce the size of the feature map and increase the number of channels. It was performed with a stride of 2. The identity mapping structure of ResNet-34 avoided the problem of gradient vanishing during gradient descent and preserved the network's deep hierarchical structure at the same time, which enabled the network to extract the higher-order image features. This guaranteed the accuracy of prediction. The final output was changed from 1000 to 2 classes to identify malignant and benign tumors. Gradient descent was performed using the Adam optimizer, and cross entropy was employed to represent the loss function. The batch size was set to 1 and the epoch to 50. The initial learning rate was set to 0.01; then, every 20 epochs, it was reduced by a factor of 10.

The proposed method was trained on a machine with NVIDIA GeForce GTX970 on an Intel i7-4770K CPU with 16 GB RAM.

2.4. *Assessment by Ophthalmologists*

To compare the classification performance between the proposed method and clinicians' visual assessment, three ophthalmologists independently reviewed all the axial CT images in the testing set. The images were anonymized before visual analysis. All ophthalmologists were blinded to the histopathological results, and the diagnosis was made based on image features including the location, number, homogeneity, and boundaries of the lesions. Then, the sensitivity, specificity, and diagnostic accuracy of the visual assessment were calculated according to the histopathological results.

2.5. Statistical Analysis

The segmentation performance of orbit mass was quantitatively assessed using dice similarity of coefficient (DSC) [35] by comparison of manual annotations and automatic segmentations. The DSC is defined as

$$DSC = 2 \times TP / (FP + 2 \times TP + FN) \quad (1)$$

where TP, FP, and FN are the numbers of true positive, false positive, and false negative detections, respectively. To visualize the automatic segmentation results, the recall-to-dice curve and the precision-to-recall curve were also drawn. Precision and recall are defined as

$$Precision = TP / (TP + FP) \quad (2)$$

$$Recall = TP / (TP + FN) \quad (3)$$

The classification performance based on DL was evaluated by the receiver operating characteristics curve (ROC) and the area under the ROC (AUC). In addition, the sensitivity, specificity, accuracy, false-positive rate, false-negative rate, positive predictive rate, and negative predictive rate of the automatic classification model and 3 ophthalmologists were calculated to further evaluate the diagnosis ability of the proposed automatic orbital tumor system.

$$Sensitivity = TP / (TP + FN) \quad (4)$$

$$Specificity = TN / (TN + FP) \quad (5)$$

$$Accuracy = (TP + TN) / (TP + TN + FP + FN) \quad (6)$$

$$False\text{-}positive\ rate = FP / (FP + TN) \quad (7)$$

$$False\text{-}negative\ rate = FN / (TP + FN) \quad (8)$$

$$Positive\ predictive\ rate = TP / (TP + FP) \quad (9)$$

$$Negative\ predictive\ rate = TN / (TN + FN) \quad (10)$$

where TP, TN, FP, and FN are the numbers of true positive, true negative, false positive, and false negative classifications.

Independent samples t-test and Chi-square test were used to analyze the differences in age and sex, respectively. The diagnostic performance of the DL-based system and 3 ophthalmologists were evaluated using the Chi-square test. All the above statistical analyses were performed using SPSS Statistics 20.0 (IBM Corporation, Armonk, NY, USA). A p value less than 0.05 was considered statistically significant. The DSC was calculated using MATLAB R2015b (The MathWorks, Natick, MA, USA). The ROC and confusion matrices were obtained with Python 3.6 using the Matplotlib package.

3. Results

3.1. Demographic Data

A total of 64 patients (mean age: 51.69 years old), including 36 males and 28 females were recruited in this study. The benign orbital tumor group consisted of 35 patients (mean age: 47.46 years old), and the malignant orbital tumor group included 29 patients (mean age: 56.79 years old). The demographic information is shown in Table 1. There were no significant differences between these two groups in terms of age and sex. Histopathological exam results showed that all patients had cavernous hemangioma in the benign orbital tumor group. In the malignant group, 25 patients (86.21%) had mucosa-associated lymphoid tissue (MLAT), 3 patients (10.34%) had diffuse large B-cell lymphoma (DLBL), and 1 patient (3.45%) had follicular lymphoma (FL).

Table 1. Demographic data of patients with orbital tumors.

Items	Total	Hemangioma	Lymphoma
Number of patients	64	35	29
Male	36	17	19
Female	28	18	10
Mean age (years)	51.69	47.46	56.79

3.2. Tumor Segmentation in CT images

A total of 69 axial CT images were randomly selected as the testing set, and this testing set was used in both segmentation and classification networks. Figure 2 shows the representative segmentation results of the benign and malignant orbital tumors using the proposed DL algorithm. Figure 2a,d show the original non-contrast-enhanced CT images of the patients with cavernous hemangioma and lymphoma, respectively. Comparison of the ground truth [red annotations in Figure 2b,e] and DL algorithm predicted segmentation [green annotations in Figure 2c,f] showed good performance in segmenting orbital tumors of different natures. The DSC quantitively described the overlap of the ground truth and the predicted result. The mean DSC value was 0.89 in the testing set. The recall-to-dice and precision-to-recall scatter diagrams in Figure 2g,h display the detailed segmentation results of all images in the testing set, demonstrating that high precision and recall were achieved in most images.

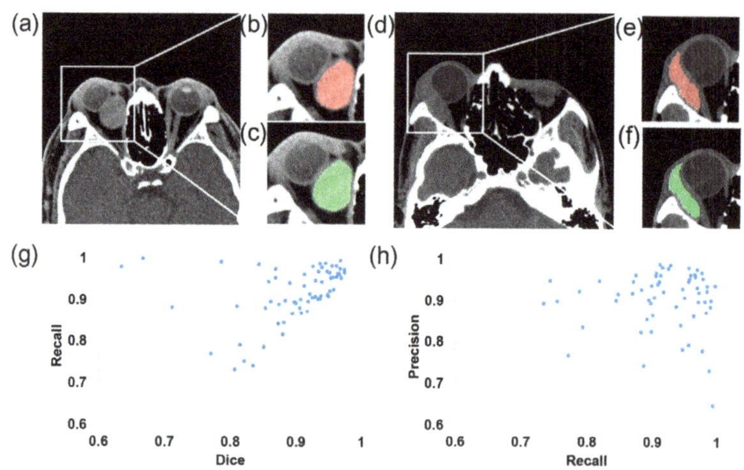

Figure 2. Segmentation performance of the deep learning algorithm: (**a**,**d**) representative original computed tomography images from patients with hemangioma and lymphoma, respectively; (**b**,**e**) manual annotations which are shown in red; (**c**,**f**) automatic segmentation results which are shown in green; (**g**,**h**) recall-to-dice and precision-to-recall scatter diagrams.

3.3. Tumor Classification

The ROC analysis demonstrates the effectiveness of ResNet-34 in benign and malignant orbital tumor classification, with an AUC of 0.9126. The diagnostic results of three ophthalmologists are also visualized in Figure 3a. Since the dataset used in this study was relatively small and from two individual institutions, 10-fold cross-validation was carried out to verify the stability and robustness of the proposed DL methods. The entire dataset of 602 images was randomly divided into 10 folds. At each passage, nine folds were randomly taken as the training set, and the remaining fold was taken as the testing set. This process was repeated 10 times to make sure each image had been trained and tested. Figure 3b shows that a consistent performance was obtained, with the AUC of the binary classification ranging from 0.8439 to 0.9546. Figure 3c–f show the confusion matrices of the DL-based model and three ophthalmologists, respectively. The number of orbital tumors that were misdiagnosed by the DL algorithm and ophthalmologist B was the same (nine images, 13.04%), which was smaller than the other ophthalmologists. There are 11 (15.94%) and 10 (14.49%) images that were misclassified by ophthalmologists A and C, respectively.

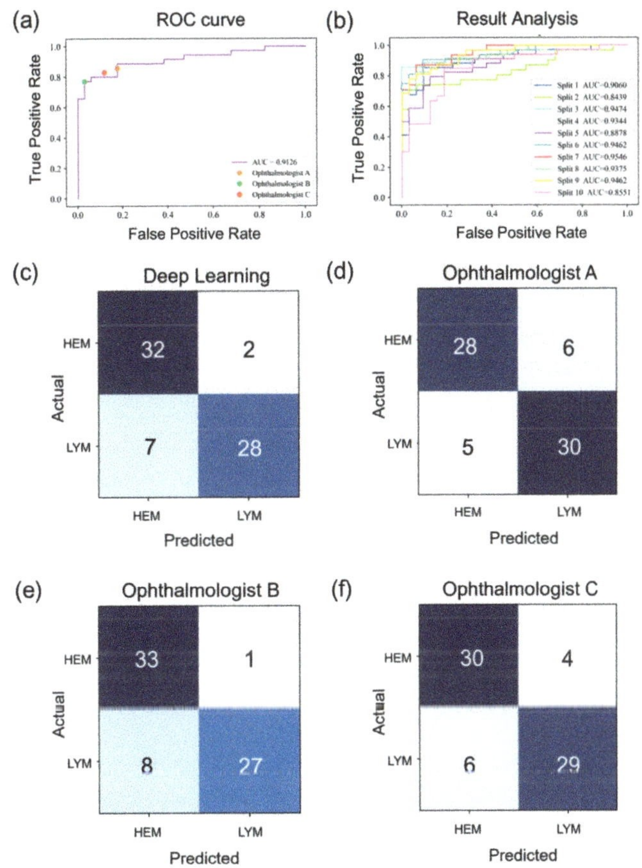

Figure 3. Classification performance of deep-learning based model and 3 ophthalmologists: (**a**) the receiver operating characteristic (ROC) curve of ResNet-34; (**b**) result analysis of the 10-fold cross-validation; (**c**–**f**) confusion matrices of the deep-learning-based model and 3 ophthalmologists.

3.4. Comparison with Ophthalmologists' Assessment

The Chi-square test showed no significant difference between the diagnostic performance of the DL-based system and three ophthalmologists ($p > 0.05$). Figure 4b displays representative examples of tumor classification. Table 2 shows that the accuracy of ResNet-34 was equal to ophthalmologist B (86.96%) and higher than ophthalmologist A (84.06%) and C (85.51%). The sensitivity of the DL-based model and three ophthalmologists was 80.00%, 85.71%, 77.14%, and 82.86%. The specificity was 94.12%, 82.35%, 97.06%, and 88.24%, respectively. Compared with ophthalmologist B, the false-negative rate of the DL algorithm was lower (20.00% versus 22.86%).

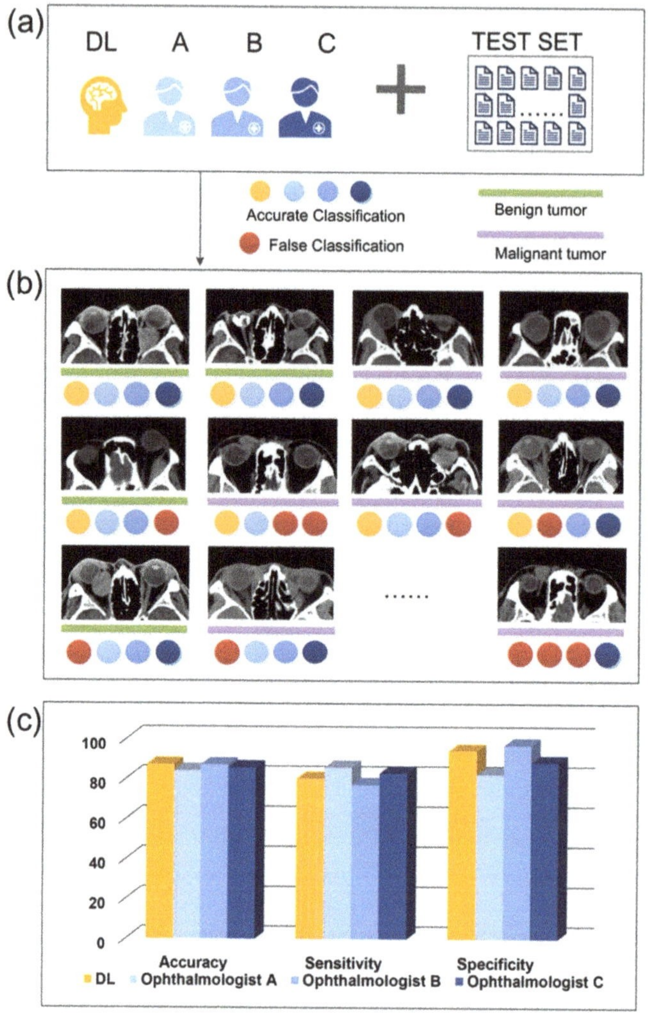

Figure 4. (**a**) Comparison of classification performance between the DL-based model and 3 ophthalmologists in the test set; (**b**) representative classification results; (**c**) comparison of the accuracy, sensitivity, and specificity of DL-based model and 3 ophthalmologists.

Table 2. Diagnostic performance of ResNet-34 and 3 ophthalmologists.

Items	ResNet-34	Ophthalmologist		
		A	B	C
Sensitivity (%)	80.00	85.71	77.14	82.86
Specificity (%)	94.12	82.35	97.06	88.24
False-Positive Rate (%)	5.88	17.65	2.94	11.76
False-Negative Rate (%)	20.00	14.29	22.86	17.14
Positive Predictive Value (%)	93.33	83.33	96.43	87.88
Negative Predictive Value (%)	82.05	84.85	80.49	83.33
Accuracy (%)	86.96	84.06	86.96	85.51
AUC	0.9126	/	/	/

4. Discussion

In this retrospective study, we established a multicenter dataset consisting of patients with cavernous hemangioma and lymphoma and proposed an end-to-end DL-based system to automatically segment and classify benign and malignant orbital tumors. The diagnostic performance of this automatic system was further explored by comparison with three certified ophthalmologists. The results showed that the automatic orbital tumor system could accurately segment orbital tumors on non-contrast-enhanced CT images with a mean DSC of 0.89. The diagnostic performance of the DL-based system was equal to three ophthalmologists.

Early recognition and diagnosis of orbital tumors are critical for treatment decisions and follow-up management. The discovery of benign tumors in orbit does not necessarily mandate its invasive treatment. A proportion of patients with asymptomatic benign orbital tumors may never require excision. Scheuerle et al. reported that all orbital hemangioma patients who received conservative treatment remained stable with a follow-up period between 3 to 10 years [3]. Patients with malignant orbital tumors may receive more aggressive treatment options, including surgery, radiotherapy, and chemotherapy [6]. A closer follow-up is also required to monitor the progress of malignant orbital tumors and ensure early intervention when recurrence is detected. Additionally, the advanced clinical stage of malignant tumors was proved to be the variable that was significantly associated with poor prognosis [36,37]. Hence, early detection of orbital tumors is also of critical importance for the prediction of prognosis.

It is often considered essential to perform a surgical orbital biopsy to confirm the diagnosis of orbital masses with unknown aetiology [38]. The surgical orbital biopsy could simultaneously be the diagnostic and therapeutic procedure for patients who need surgical excision due to visual threat or suspicion of malignancy. Nevertheless, for patients with benign orbital tumors that can be managed conservatively, this invasive procedure could merely be used as a diagnostic criterion. In these cases, the accuracy of non-invasive or minimally invasive diagnostic modalities should be improved.

CT and MRI, exhibiting the location, content, soft tissue, and bone characteristics of orbital tumors, are important tools to assist ophthalmologists in making the preliminary diagnosis. However, the accuracy of clinical and radiological diagnosis was not always satisfactory, and the positive prediction rate relied highly on the skills and knowledge of the reviewers. Koukkoulli et al. [39] retrospectively analyzed patients who underwent surgical orbital biopsy from 2003 to 2015, involving more than 100 orbital lesions. The accuracy of the diagnoses made by the ophthalmologists and the radiologists was compared with histological results. The results showed that correct diagnoses were reached in less than 50% of all cases reviewed by ophthalmologists and radiologists alike. In addition, 34.8% and 39.3% of all cases reviewed by ophthalmologists and radiologists reported no differential diagnosis. In practical clinical settings, ophthalmologists often asked a detailed history and performed a comprehensive ocular examination, and then correctly concluded that orbital imaging was required but reached no specific diagnosis. Radiologists often reported the imaging findings using suggestive language and provided a list of possible diagnoses. In our study, the accuracy of differentiating benign and malignant orbital tumors reached 86.96%, exhibiting the robustness of the proposed system. The AUC of 10-fold cross-validation ranged from 0.8439 to 0.9546, which indicated the stability and repeatability of this DL-based system.

To differentiate benign and malignant orbital tumors, several studies attempted to interpret CT and/or MRI to figure out predictive features, but the results were not always consistent. Ben et al. [17] established a guideline for reviewing orbital CT and/or MRI based on 84 features. Applying this guideline, three physicians reevaluated all images. Then, the differential ability of the multiple features to discriminate between benign, malignant, and inflammatory orbital lesions was calculated. None of these features had the high sensitivity to distinguish the nature of different orbital lesions. Xian et al. [10] reported that some MRI image features were associated with malignant orbital lesions, and the inter-observer agreement between the two observers was excellent. The features that had a high sensitivity and specificity for the prediction of malignant lesions were the involvement of preseptal space, ill-defined margin, molding around orbital structures, isointensity on T2-weighted MRI images, homogeneous enhancement, and washout-type time-intensity curve (TIC). Yuan et al. [40] further explored the diagnostic efficacy of TIC on dynamic contrast-enhanced MRI images. The results demonstrated that the orbital mass with a washout pattern of TIC may be more likely to be malignant, while those having the persistent pattern of TIC would be more suggestive to be identified as benign. In addition, Khalek et al. [41] found that the apparent diffusion coefficient value at three-T diffusion MRI was a feature that could diagnose malignant versus benign orbital lesions.

The aforementioned studies indicated that features of benign and malignant orbital masses may be overlapped, and it may be difficult to establish an efficient feature map. Furthermore, the detection and annotation of orbital lesions were still manual. Some features, such as the shape and margin of masses, were assessed by ophthalmologists or radiologists. Such processes with human involvement may be influenced by the experience of the reviewer. The lack of ophthalmologists [42] and the increased workload of radiologists [43] make it even harder to accurate diagnosis of benign and malignant orbital tumors. In this study, the proposed end-to-end orbital tumor diagnosis system applied the algorithm to automatically analyze the high-level features of non-contrast-enhanced CT, discerning malignant from benign tumors without any manual processing.

AI-based models could help improve the precision of image interpretation. Several studies had showed the efficiency of AI-based algorithms in distinguishing orbital masses on CT and MRI. Guo et al. [27] employed an MR-based radiomics signature to distinguish ocular adnexal lymphoma (OAL) and idiopathic orbital inflammation (IOI), which reached an AUC of 0.74 and 0.73 in primary and validation cohorts. Han et al. [44] used an ML-based model to automatically identify the differences in orbital cavernous venous malformation from non-contrast-enhanced CT. Hou et al. [28] reported a bag-of-features (BOF)-based radiomic analysis method, with a support vector machine as the classifier. Differentiation with augmentation achieved an AUC of 0.803 in the test group from contrast-enhanced MRI, but the same analysis results from pre-contrast MRI were significantly less reliable. Radiomics has the advantage of extracting and analyzing high-dimensional quantitative features obtained from medical images at high throughput [45]. However, the efficacy of radiomics-based methods relied on the segmentation accuracy of the ROI, the quantity and type of extracted features, and the choice of the classifier. In the studies mentioned above, ROI segmentation was conducted manually, which may be affected by the subjective bias of observers. Bi et al. [46] applied three DL models to differentiate cavernous hemangiomas from schwannomas. The first two models were employed for eye and tumor location. The third classification model had an accuracy of 91.13% in the transverse T1 CE sequence. However, the highest accuracies were achieved in CE MRI, an invasive imaging examination. In this study, we simplified the workflow. In the testing set, after inputting non-contrast-enhanced CT images, the DL-based system could segment the tumoral regions and output the diagnosis of benign and malignant orbital tumors end-to-end, reducing the workload of clinicians.

Although the present study demonstrated the potential utility of DL in the detection and classification of orbital tumors, it had several limitations. First, the number of patients included was relatively small. For further studies, a larger number of cases and more types of orbital tumors are necessary. Second, in this retrospective study, the CT images selected had different slice thicknesses and scanning parameters with different CT scanners. However, these differences of input data also demonstrated the generalizability of the proposed method. Third, although the diagnosis performance reached a satisfactory result that was equal to three certified ophthalmologists, it was not compared with contrast-enhanced CT or MRI images. Therefore, it is promising to use different kinds of input images and make comparisons between CT and MRI images, as well as between non-contrast-enhanced and contrast-enhanced images. Fourth, the axial CT scans used in this study could only provide two-dimensional tumor features. In the future, location features should be combined with three-dimensional medical images to improve the diagnosis performance of automatic orbital tumor analysis systems.

5. Conclusions

In conclusion, the results of our study showed that the proposed DL-based system could effectively segment and classify different orbital tumors. It may provide accurate diagnostic assistance for inexperienced clinicians and help make treatment decisions. In the future, with the improvement of DL technology, these techniques have the potential to assist in the diagnosis of different tumors in several bodily areas.

Author Contributions: Conceptualization, J.S., J.Z., W.G. and J.Y.; methodology, K.J. and X.G.; software, Y.X.; validation, T.J. and C.W.; formal analysis, X.X.; investigation, J.S., J.Z. and Y.X.; resources, J.S. and T.J.; data curation, X.G., X.X. and F.S.; writing—original draft preparation, J.S. and J.Z.; writing—review and editing, K.J., W.G. and J.Y.; visualization, K.S.; supervision, W.G. and J.Y.; project administration, W.G. and J.Y.; funding acquisition, W.G. and J.Y. All authors have read and agreed to the published version of the manuscript.

Funding: This research was funded by the National Key Research and Development Program of China, grant number 2019YFC0118400, National Natural Science Foundation Regional Innovation and Development Joint Fund, grant number U20A20386, National Natural Science Foundation of China, grant number 61975178, Key research and development program of Zhejiang Province, grant number 2019C03020, Natural Science Foundation of Zhejiang Province, grant number LR20F050002.

Institutional Review Board Statement: The study was conducted in accordance with the Declaration of Helsinki, and approved by the Institutional Review Board of The Second Affiliated Hospital of Zhejiang University (Approval Code: 2020-476, and date of approval: 9 June 2020) and Tianjin Medical University Eye Hospital (Approval Code: 2018KY57, and date of approval: 31 December 2018).

Informed Consent Statement: The request for the waiver of patient informed consent have been approved by t the Institutional Review Board of The Second Affiliated Hospital of Zhejiang University and Tianjin Medical University Eye Hospital. Patient consent was waived due to retrospective nature of this study, in which identification information in computed tomography images was removed from all participants.

Data Availability Statement: The data presented in this study are available on request from the corresponding author. The data are not publicly available due to privacy issue.

Acknowledgments: The authors would like to acknowledge Xiaoling Huang and Xindi Liu (Department of Ophthalmology, the Second Affiliated Hospital of Zhejiang University, School of Medicine) for their intellectual contributions to reviewing orbital CT images and making diagnoses.

Conflicts of Interest: The authors declare no conflict of interest.

References

1. Shields, J.A.; Shields, C.L.; Scartozzi, R. Survey of 1264 patients with orbital tumors and simulating lesions—The 2002 montgomery lecture, part 1. *Ophthalmology* **2004**, *111*, 997–1008. [CrossRef] [PubMed]
2. Rootman, D.B.; Heran, M.K.; Rootman, J.; White, V.A.; Luemsamran, P.; Yucel, Y.H. Cavernous venous malformations of the orbit (so-called cavernous haemangioma): A comprehensive evaluation of their clinical, imaging and histologic nature. *Br. J. Ophthalmol.* **2014**, *98*, 880–888. [CrossRef] [PubMed]
3. Scheuerle, A.F.; Steiner, H.H.; Kolling, G.; Kunze, S.; Aschoff, A. Treatment and long-term outcome of patients with orbital cavernomas. *Am. J. Ophthalmol.* **2004**, *138*, 237–244. [CrossRef] [PubMed]
4. Harris, G.J. Cavernous hemangioma of the orbital apex: Pathogenetic considerations in surgical management. *Am. J. Ophthalmol.* **2010**, *150*, 764–773. [CrossRef] [PubMed]
5. Low, C.M.; Stokken, J.K. Typical orbital pathologies: Hemangioma. *J. Neurol. Surg. B Skull Base* **2021**, *82*, 20–26. [CrossRef] [PubMed]
6. Woolf, D.K.; Ahmed, M.; Plowman, P.N. Primary lymphoma of the ocular adnexa (orbital lymphoma) and primary intraocular lymphoma. *Clin. Oncol.* **2012**, *24*, 339–344. [CrossRef] [PubMed]
7. Kharod, S.M.; Herman, M.P.; Morris, C.G.; Lightsey, J.; Mendenhall, W.M.; Mendenhall, N.P. Radiotherapy in the management of orbital lymphoma a single institution's experience over 4 decades. *Am. J. Clin. Oncol.-Cancer Clin. Trials* **2018**, *41*, 100–106.

8. Demirci, H.; Shields, C.L.; Shields, J.A.; Honavar, S.G.; Mercado, G.J.; Tovilla, J.C. Orbital tumors in the older adult population. *Ophthalmology* **2002**, *109*, 243–248. [CrossRef]
9. Khan, S.N.; Sepahdari, A.R. Orbital masses: CT and MRI of common vascular lesions, benign tumors, and malignancies. *Saudi. J Ophthalmol.* **2012**, *26*, 373–383. [CrossRef]
10. Xian, J.F.; Zhang, Z.Y.; Wang, Z.C.; Li, J.; Yang, B.T.; Man, F.Y.; Chang, Q.L.; Zhang, Y.T. Value of MR imaging in the differentiation of benign and malignant orbital tumors in adults. *Eur. Radiol.* **2010**, *20*, 1692–1702. [CrossRef]
11. Zhang, L.; Li, X.; Tang, F.; Gan, L.; Wei, X. Diagnostic imaging methods and comparative analysis of orbital cavernous hemangioma. *Front. Oncol.* **2020**, *10*, 577452. [CrossRef]
12. Russell, E.J.; Czervionke, L.; Huckman, M.; Daniels, D.; McLachlan, D. Ct of the inferomedial orbit and the lacrimal drainage apparatus: Normal and pathologic anatomy. *AJR Am. J. Roentgenol.* **1985**, *145*, 1147–1154. [CrossRef]
13. Langer, B.G.; Mafee, M.F.; Pollack, S.; Spigos, D.G.; Gyi, B. Mri of the normal orbit and optic pathway. *Radiol. Clin. N. Am.* **1987**, *25*, 429–446. [CrossRef]
14. Joseph, A.K.; Guerin, J.B.; Eckel, L.J.; Dalvin, L.A.; Keating, G.F.; Liebo, G.B.; Benson, J.C.; Brinjikji, W.; Laack, N.N.; Silvera, V.M. Imaging findings of pediatric orbital masses and tumor mimics. *Radiographics* **2022**, *42*, 880–897. [CrossRef]
15. Priego, G.; Majos, C.; Climent, F.; Muntane, A. Orbital lymphoma: Imaging features and differential diagnosis. *Insights. Imaging* **2012**, *3*, 337–344. [CrossRef]
16. Beckett, K.R.; Moriarity, A.K.; Langer, J.M. Safe use of contrast media: What the radiologist needs to know. *Radiographics* **2015**, *35*, 1738–1750. [CrossRef]
17. Ben Simon, G.J.; Annunziata, C.C.; Fink, J.; Villablanca, P.; McCann, J.D.; Goldberg, R.A. Rethinking orbital imaging—Establishing guidelines for interpreting orbital imaging studies and evaluating their predictive value in patients with orbital tumors. *Ophthalmology* **2005**, *112*, 2196–2207. [CrossRef]
18. Nichols, J.A.; Herbert Chan, H.W.; Baker, M.A.B. Machine learning: Applications of artificial intelligence to imaging and diagnosis. *Biophys. Rev.* **2019**, *11*, 111–118. [CrossRef]
19. Cho, S.M.; Austin, P.C.; Ross, H.J.; Abdel-Qadir, H.; Chicco, D.; Tomlinson, G.; Taheri, C.; Foroutan, F.; Lawler, P.R.; Billia, F.; et al. Machine learning compared with conventional statistical models for predicting myocardial infarction readmission and mortality: A systematic review. *Can. J. Cardiol.* **2021**, *37*, 1207–1214. [CrossRef]
20. Brehar, R.; Mitrea, D.A.; Vancea, F.; Marita, T.; Nedevschi, S.; Lupsor-Platon, M.; Rotaru, M.; Badea, R.I. Comparison of deep-learning and conventional machine-learning methods for the automatic recognition of the hepatocellular carcinoma areas from ultrasound images. *Sensors* **2020**, *20*, 3085. [CrossRef]
21. Ye, Y.; Xiong, Y.; Zhou, Q.; Wu, J.; Li, X.; Xiao, X. Comparison of machine learning methods and conventional logistic regressions for predicting gestational diabetes using routine clinical data: A retrospective cohort study. *J. Diabetes. Res.* **2020**, *2020*, 4168340. [CrossRef] [PubMed]
22. Ting, D.S.W.; Cheung, C.Y.L.; Lim, G.; Tan, G.S.W.; Quang, N.D.; Gan, A.; Hamzah, H.; Garcia-Franco, R.; San Yeo, I.Y.; Lee, S.Y.; et al. Development and validation of a deep learning system for diabetic retinopathy and related eye diseases using retinal images from multiethnic populations with diabetes. *JAMA* **2017**, *318*, 2211–2223. [CrossRef] [PubMed]
23. Ting, D.S.W.; Pasquale, L.R.; Peng, L.; Campbell, J.P.; Lee, A.Y.; Raman, R.; Tan, G.S.W.; Schmetterer, L.; Keane, P.A.; Wong, T.Y. Artificial intelligence and deep learning in ophthalmology. *Br. J. Ophthalmol.* **2019**, *103*, 167–175. [CrossRef] [PubMed]
24. Bao, X.-L.; Sun, Y.-J.; Zhan, X.; Li, G.-Y. Orbital and eyelid diseases: The next breakthrough in artificial intelligence? *Front. Cell. Dev. Biol.* **2022**, *10*, 1069248. [CrossRef]
25. Pan, L.; Chen, K.; Zheng, Z.; Zhao, Y.; Yang, P.; Li, Z.; Wu, S. Aging of chinese bony orbit: Automatic calculation based on UNet++ and connected component analysis. *Surg. Radiol. Anat.* **2022**, *44*, 749–758. [CrossRef]
26. Li, Z.; Chen, K.; Yang, J.; Pan, L.; Wang, Z.; Yang, P.; Wu, S.; Li, J. Deep learning-based ct radiomics for feature representation and analysis of aging characteristics of asian bony orbit. *J. Craniofac. Surg.* **2022**, *33*, 312–318. [CrossRef]
27. Guo, J.; Liu, Z.; Shen, C.; Li, Z.; Yan, F.; Tian, J.; Xian, J. Mr-based radiomics signature in differentiating ocular adnexal lymphoma from idiopathic orbital inflammation. *Eur. Radiol.* **2018**, *28*, 3872–3881. [CrossRef]
28. Hou, Y.; Xie, X.; Chen, J.; Lv, P.; Jiang, S.; He, X.; Yang, L.; Zhao, F. Bag-of-features-based radiomics for differentiation of ocular adnexal lymphoma and idiopathic orbital inflammation from contrast-enhanced mri. *Eur. Radiol.* **2021**, *31*, 24–33. [CrossRef]
29. Hua, K.-L.; Hsu, C.-H.; Hidayati, H.C.; Cheng, W.-H.; Chen, Y.-J. Computer-aided classification of lung nodules on computed tomography images via deep learning technique. *Onco Targets Ther.* **2015**, *8*, 2015–2022.
30. Nam, J.G.; Park, S.; Hwang, E.J.; Lee, J.H.; Jin, K.-N.; Lim, K.Y.; Vu, T.H.; Sohn, J.H.; Hwang, S.; Goo, J.M.; et al. Development and validation of deep learning-based automatic detection algorithm for malignant pulmonary nodules on chest radiographs. *Radiology* **2019**, *290*, 218–228. [CrossRef]
31. Gao, X.W.; Hui, R.; Tian, Z. Classification of ct brain images based on deep learning networks. *Comput. Methods Programs Biomed.* **2017**, *138*, 49–56. [CrossRef]
32. Balkenende, L.; Teuwen, J.; Mann, R.M. Application of deep learning in breast cancer imaging. *Semin. Nucl. Med.* **2022**, *52*, 584–596. [CrossRef]
33. Yin, X.X.; Sun, L.; Fu, Y.; Lu, R.; Zhang, Y. U-net-based medical image segmentation. *J. Healthc. Eng.* **2022**, *2022*, 4189781. [CrossRef]

34. He, K.; Zhang, X.; Ren, S.; Sun, J. Deep residual learning for image recognition. In Proceedings of the 2016 IEEE Conference on Computer Vision and Pattern Recognition (CVPR), Seattle, WA, USA, 27–30 June 2016.
35. Dice, L.R. Measures of the amount of ecologic association between species. *Ecology* **1945**, *26*, 297–302. [CrossRef]
36. Hsu, C.R.; Chen, Y.Y.; Yao, M.; Wei, Y.H.; Hsieh, Y.T.; Liao, S.L. Orbital and ocular adnexal lymphoma: A review of epidemiology and prognostic factors in Taiwan. *Eye* **2021**, *35*, 1946–1953. [CrossRef]
37. Olsen, T.G.; Heegaard, S. Orbital lymphoma. *Surv. Ophthalmol.* **2019**, *64*, 45–66. [CrossRef]
38. Mombaerts, I.; Ramberg, I.; Coupland, S.E.; Heegaard, S. Diagnosis of orbital mass lesions: Clinical, radiological, and pathological recommendations. *Surv. Ophthalmol.* **2019**, *64*, 741–756. [CrossRef]
39. Koukkoulli, A.; Pilling, J.D.; Patatas, K.; El-Hindy, N.; Chang, B.; Kalantzis, G. How accurate is the clinical and radiological evaluation of orbital lesions in comparison to surgical orbital biopsy? *Eye* **2018**, *32*, 1329–1333. [CrossRef]
40. Yuan, Y.; Kuai, X.P.; Chen, X.S.; Tao, X.F. Assessment of dynamic contrast-enhanced magnetic resonance imaging in the differentiation of malignant from benign orbital masses. *Eur. J. Radiol.* **2013**, *82*, 1506–1511. [CrossRef]
41. Khalek, A.A.; Razek, A.; Elkhamary, S.; Mousa, A. Differentiation between benign and malignant orbital tumors at 3-T diffusion mr-imaging. *Neuroradiology* **2011**, *53*, 517–522.
42. Resnikoff, S.; Felch, W.; Gauthier, T.M.; Spivey, B. The number of ophthalmologists in practice and training worldwide: A growing gap despite more than 200,000 practitioners. *Br. J. Ophthalmol.* **2012**, *96*, 783–787. [CrossRef] [PubMed]
43. Bruls, R.J.M.; Kwee, R.M. Workload for radiologists during on-call hours: Dramatic increase in the past 15 years. *Insights Imaging* **2020**, *11*, 121. [CrossRef] [PubMed]
44. Han, Q.; Du, L.; Mo, Y.; Huang, C.; Yuan, Q. Machine learning based non-enhanced ct radiomics for the identification of orbital cavernous venous malformations: An innovative tool. *J. Craniofac. Surg.* **2022**, *33*, 814–820. [CrossRef] [PubMed]
45. Lambin, P.; Rios-Velazquez, E.; Leijenaar, R.; Carvalho, S.; van Stiphout, R.G.; Granton, P.; Zegers, C.M.; Gillies, R.; Boellard, R.; Dekker, A.; et al. Radiomics: Extracting more information from medical images using advanced feature analysis. *Eur. J. Cancer.* **2012**, *48*, 441–446. [CrossRef] [PubMed]
46. Bi, S.; Chen, R.; Zhang, K.; Xiang, Y.; Wang, R.; Lin, H.; Yang, H. Differentiate cavernous hemangioma from schwannoma with artificial intelligence (AI). *Ann. Transl. Med.* **2020**, *8*, 710. [CrossRef]

MDPI
St. Alban-Anlage 66
4052 Basel
Switzerland
Tel. +41 61 683 77 34
Fax +41 61 302 89 18
www.mdpi.com

Journal of Personalized Medicine Editorial Office
E-mail: jpm@mdpi.com
www.mdpi.com/journal/jpm